SMALL
STEPS
BIG
CHANGE

From Burnout
to Balance

———————

To all the dedicated health professional and frontline workers who worked so hard for the benefit of so many during the global COVID-19 pandemic of 2020.

———————

From Burnout to Balance

HOW TO RECLAIM YOUR LIFE
& IMPROVE YOUR HEALTH

Harriet Griffey

Hardie Grant

BOOKS

Contents

Introduction
.... 07

01

Signs & Symptoms of Burnout

Quick checklist
.... 19

Identifying the problem
.... 23

The limbic system
.... 29

Feel-good hormones
.... 33

Inflammation
.... 39

Quiz: How close are you to burnout
.... 47

02

Be Stress Smart

What is stress?
.... 55

Breathe
.... 59

Connect
.... 63

Increasing resilience
.... 67

Managing uncertainty
.... 71

Living mindfully
.... 75

When to ask for help
.... 81

03

Workplace Stress

Your workplace
.... 89

Environment
.... 95

Colleagues
.... 97

Expectations
.... 101

04

Social Media Stress

Social Media
.... 107

Continuous Partial Attention (CPA)
.... 109

Discontent
.... 113

Cutting back
.... 115

Watching the news
.... 119

05

24-hour Crisis Plan

Crisis point
.... 125

Key signs
.... 127

First steps
.... 129

Burnout first aid
.... 130

06

Four weeks to recover your life

Altering your baseline
.... 135

Work life
.... 139

Sleep well
.... 145

Eat smart
.... 151

Exercise & play
.... 159

Conclusion

.... 165

Appendix
.... 170

About the author
.... 172

Index
.... 174

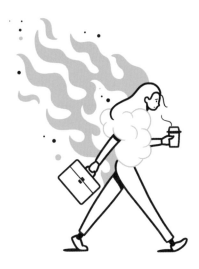

Introduction

Burnout. A recent headline in the UK's *Guardian* newspaper called it 'a sinister and insidious epidemic' and went on to document the growing awareness of this sort of work-related stress, which can result in psychological and physical breakdown.

In May 2020, CNBC reported that Google's CEO Sundar Pichai asked employees to take time off to address work-from-home burnout, in acknowledgement of the adjustment needed as the world's workforce continued in coronavirus lockdown. Bloomberg Businessweek also reported on 'pandemic-induced burnout' as juggling full-time work with additional family responsibilities, the stress of confinement and concern about family and friends from whom we had to remain separate, became longer term. The continuous uncertainty (see page 71) of when restrictions might end, and the long-term impact on lives and livelihoods of these, was another anxiety. The relentless bad-news cycle didn't help either.

Sheryl Sandburg, CEO of Facebook, writing an op-ed for Fortune magazine on May 7th 2020 cited research that showed a particular burden was being felt by working women, placing them at greater risk. "The coronavirus is creating a 'double double shift' for women," she wrote. "According to recent surveys by LeanIn.org and Survey Monkey conducted in April, one in four women say they are experiencing severe anxiety with physical symptoms like a racing heartbeat. One in 10 men say the same. More than half of all women are currently struggling with sleep issues."

Working from home affected many struggling to adapt to intense Zoom meetings and being constantly online, but for frontline staff and healthcare professionals there was the additional stress of increased workload under siege conditions. Organisations like the Society of Critical Care Medicine (for intensive care professionals) in the US were quick to recognise this and produced their own guidelines. These were designed to define burnout, identify risk factors, review signs and symptoms, examine ways to help prevent burnout and then, crucially, formulate a plan to manage staff. Recognised as a very real issue, burnout became a feature of many pandemic discussions.

'You cannot be at peak performance forever,' António Horta-Osorio told the BBC in early 2020. In 2011, the banker took eight weeks off work to recuperate after dealing with the fallout of the financial crisis at the bank for which he was responsible. Having turned its financial performance around, today he is CEO of Lloyds Banking Group and a big proponent of safeguarding ourselves against burnout. 'It's really important to combine peak performance with periods of rest, so you can recover,' he said. 'You also have to have holidays in order to think about different things and regenerate your body and mind.'

It turns out, though, that we're really bad at taking time off – even on holiday. Research by YouGov in 2018 found that 60 per cent of those on holiday still checked their work emails, and this seems a global trend. One of the downsides to our constant technological connectivity is that, just because it's possible to work 24/7, we somehow feel obliged to do so. Very few of us will deliberately switch off our work connections, even when on holiday. Some people even claim that it is more stressful to log out than it is to keep working.

We seem to have become incapable of doing nothing, despite the fact that taking time out can actually enhance creativity and its sidekick, productivity. Allowing the brain to idle in neutral, indulging in a daydream or even feeling bored have all become alien concepts. Now, though, many of us are learning the hard way that we need to rebalance our lives, and burnout is often the price paid for that knowledge.

WHO classification

The World Health Organisation's International Classification of Diseases (ICD-10), first endorsed in 1990, identifies burnout as a 'state of vital exhaustion' and lists it as related to life-management difficulties. In 2019, WHO's updated ICD-11 described burnout as:

- feelings of energy depletion or exhaustion;
- increased mental distance from one's job, or feelings of negativism or cynicism related to one's job;
- reduced professional efficacy.

For those who've experienced it, there can be no doubt that the effects of burnout are life-changing, and recovery takes time. When we are approaching burnout, however, it can sometimes be hard to identify the early warning signs.

"Everyone told me to be careful. 'Watch out: you're burning the candle at both ends.' 'Maybe you could do with some support?' And I would wave them away dismissively. Of course I could cope. They hadn't seen anything yet. So I sailed on, hitting target after target, making my company more successful than it had ever been, until suddenly I couldn't do it anymore. I couldn't get out of bed some days, and when I did, I couldn't stand up, walk in a straight line or talk sense. I felt physically sick in the presence of colleagues; I couldn't make decisions, take notes or sit in meetings."

ANONYMOUS, *The Guardian*, 22 July 2017

The Maslach Burnout Inventory

Burnout even has its own test, the Maslach Burnout Inventory (MBI). This was devised in 1981 and is used in occupational health, so, contrary to some claims, burnout is not a modern phenomenon invented by 'Generation Snowflake'. In fact, it's often 'Generation Sandwich' – those sandwiched between caring for children and ageing parents, while also trying to juggle peak career stress – that can be most at risk. Burnout typically affects those of us trying to be all things to all people. As the warning signs can also resemble depression – and it's not difficult to see how the two might be related – it's sometimes hard to spot early signs. When we get caught in long-term patterns of stress, we adapt to the constantly elevated levels of stress hormones. It begins to feel 'normal' to be functioning like this: strung out, unable to concentrate, wired. It takes time – weeks, sometimes – to reset our internal stress thermostat to a healthy baseline.

The difference between coping and not coping is highly individual and very slim. Symptoms of burnout may be low-key at first, but their cumulative effect is insidious, building over time until the final straw overwhelms us.

Tiredness – the sort that creates feelings of emotional, mental and physical exhaustion that is unrelieved by sleep – is an early warning signal. Sleep becomes problematic: we may have difficulties falling asleep, or a tendency to wake very early in the morning with a racing mind and pounding heart (those stress hormones again). Another sign can be the sense that we're on a treadmill, that what we're doing isn't good enough and is ineffective or never-ending, whether this is studying, work, or parenting. Finally, we may experience an increasing sense of being cut off from ourselves and other people, a sort of dissociation that starts to affect our closest relationships.

Contrary to what we might think, there is not one particular group or demographic that's more at risk than another. There's been some criticism of millennials in recent years, accusing them of being 'snowflakes' who have no resilience and don't know the reality of hard work, but the reality is somewhat different. In 2016, a report from the Manpower Group discovered that, contrary to the idea that millennials (who now make up a third of the global workforce) are lazy, they are actually working as hard, if not harder, than other generations. Seventy-three per cent report working more than 40 hours a week, and nearly a quarter work more than 50 hours. Millennials from the Indian subcontinent claim the longest working week and Australia the shortest (on average, 52 and 41 hours a week respectively), while 26 per cent globally are working two or more paid jobs.

What's happening?

When the pressure is on, the nervous system responds by churning out lots of adrenaline and cortisol. These are compensatory stress hormones designed to help us cope and keep going – in the short term. Maintaining this state over the long term is really not good for our body or minds. The adrenal glands that produce these hormones become relentlessly over-stimulated and can become damaged and unpredictable, sometimes failing to produce enough hormones on demand, sometimes over-producing them, leaving us feeling alternatively completely floored and depleted or wired and panicky.

Understanding how your body responds, what causes its stress reaction and what this feels like will help you to notice those signs that are really a red alert, and respond to them before the situation becomes catastrophic. This understanding is vital if we are to reverse or prevent burnout.

"According to the World Health Organisation, burnout has three elements: feelings of exhaustion, mental detachment from one's job and poorer performance at work. But waiting until you're already fully burned out to do something about it doesn't help at all – and you wouldn't wait to treat any other illness until it was too late."

BBC WORKLIFE, June 2019

That's the problem with burnout: it tends to creep up on us unawares. We do manage, often by burning the candle at both ends, to stay on top of impossible schedules for sustained periods of time. We pride ourselves on being able to multitask, producing that 5,000-word report *and* a batch of cupcakes for the school bake sale, and never missing a work deadline or a school function, even when the only time off we get is at 3 a.m. (*after* the cat's litter tray has been cleaned). Then we kid ourselves that we can manage on four hours' sleep a night as we haul ourselves out of bed for a 7 a.m. spin class. Zero-hours contracts, the gig economy, job insecurity and financial concerns don't feature too highly on our favourite Instagram accounts, and we can end up feeling ashamed for struggling (see page 20). If any of this is ringing a bell, it may be that your work–life balance needs re-evaluating, because the impact of trying to function like this for days, weeks or even months on end will take its toll.

Heart problems

Burnout is not only bad for our mental health, but our physical health too. A 2020 study published in the *European Journal of Preventive Cardiology* found that those with the highest levels of burnout had a 20 per cent higher risk of developing atrial fibrillation (AF), a heart condition that causes an irregular and often abnormally fast heart rate. According to lead researcher Dr Parveen Garg, 'Vital exhaustion, commonly referred to as burnout syndrome, is typically caused by prolonged and profound stress at work or home.' The study surveyed more than 11,000 people over a 25-year period and, while further research is needed, Dr Garg believes that the two main reasons burnout causes AF are the heightened and prolonged activation of the body's stress response and increased inflammation (see page 39). When these two things are constantly triggered over a long period, they can have serious and damaging effects on heart tissue, which is what could eventually lead to the development of AF. This in turn increases the risk of heart attack and strokes.

Fertility problems

Stress hormones tend to have an impact on other hormones. For women, this can play havoc with their menstrual cycle. Periods can become irregular and less frequent, as a stressed-out body will prioritise survival over reproduction. It may take some time for irregular periods to regularise and for a woman's ovulation cycle to improve, even after a healthy life balance has been restored. If this is you and you are struggling to conceive, every recommendation to avoid or recover from burnout made in this book will help improve chances of conception. Chronic stress can have an impact on libido, and without a regular sex life, the chances are reduced even further.

The long-term impact of burnout

Over time, the impact of prioritising the survival response – which is what an acute stress response is – may deplete all other body systems, including the immune system. This makes the chances of minor illness like coughs and colds much more likely, as well as more serious illnesses like chronic fatigue syndrome (CFS) or myalgic encephalomyelitis (ME), and autoimmune disorders like lupus and rheumatoid arthritis. A worst-case scenario of complete burnout, with is really the final stage of the vital exhaustion as described by WHO, can increase these risks. And when that happens, it's mostly because we either missed or ignored the warning signs. The smart thing to do is to pay attention to those early warnings and take steps to restore the balance our lives need to avoid it.

01

·

Signs &
Symptoms
of Burnout

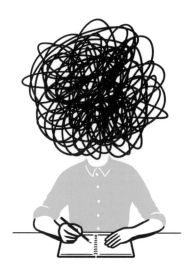

Quick Checklist

How do you know whether what you're experiencing might be symptoms of burnout?

Do you feel permanently exhausted, wrung out, trapped, angry and dissociated? Do you feel you are working harder and longer but achieving less? Do you constantly feel under the weather, or suffer from persistent aches, pains, niggles and minor illnesses that won't go away?

Can you tick these three boxes without a second's hesitation?

- Emotional, mental and/or physical exhaustion
  that isn't alleviated by sleeping .... ☐
- An increasing sense of being cut off from
  yourself and from other people .... ☐
- Feeling that you are less effective at doing what you've
  always done, either at work or at home .... ☐

If you feel you've reached this stage, burnout isn't just an emotional state: there's also a significant physical effect on your health. One will impact on the other, affecting how you feel both physically and emotionally. Living in a constant state of low-level stress, with an increasing reliance on your stress hormones to keep you going, can lead to adrenal exhaustion. If you reach a point of total collapse, it takes a long time to come back from.

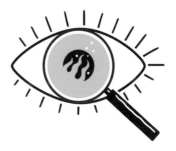

Identifying the Problem

One of the difficulties with burnout is that its build-up can be very gradual. It's all too easy to hit crisis point without realising that this is where we've been headed for weeks, if not for months or years. This is because the human body (and mind) is a marvel of adaptation and will, in time, adapt so well to a state of continuous low-grade stress that it begins to feel normal, even while we're heading towards burnout.

When we are faced with a stressful situation, the resources we need to manage it will rev up; but once the stressful situation has resolved, our body should then return to its baseline, resting state. However, if we subject ourselves to relentless stress that continuously activates and re-activates our stress response, that baseline moves to a new place of adaptation. But this is actually a place of *maladaptation*, because it's not how we are designed to function in the long term. The damage this may do, and how long it will take to kick in, is difficult to assess because we are all different. However, if we continue down this path it will become unsustainable, the cracks will show, and eventually the dam will break.

"All those years reading Camus, Sartre and Hamsun and still I had failed to see the signs stacking up over the previous months: the rising sense of panic, the narcolepsy-like bouts of sleep at inopportune moments, the way my digestive system went into revolt. There were puking jags, migraines and aching muscles. Food lost its flavour and noises became amplified, so much so that I became fixated on a neighbour's cockerel that crowed every morning from 3.55am, and which I wanted to strangle. Even the chimes of the local church bells sounded malevolent, as if mocking my shortcomings."

BENJAMIN MYERS, *The Guardian*, 3 January 2020

'Vital exhaustion'

This is the term coined by Dr Parveen Garg to describe the exhaustion of our life-giving body systems. When the pressure is on, the nervous system responds. The hypothalamus in the brain registers this and alerts the pituitary gland which, in turn, switches the adrenals on to full power. This activation of the HPA axis means that levels of stress hormones adrenaline (epinephrine) and cortisol, and neurotransmitter noradrenaline (norepinephrine), are revved up in a way that's designed to keep you going – in the short term – while you are deprived of sleep, regular food and time to rest. This is a feature of the body's fight/flight/freeze response to threat. What's crucial about this response is that it's designed *for the short term*, to give us the resources we need to get out of danger and enable us to survive. Maintaining this acutely reactive state in the long term is not what the body was designed to do, and in time its insidious effect is detrimental to body and mind.

Over time, the adrenal glands that produce these hormones become hyper-stimulated and unpredictable, sometimes failing to produce enough hormones on demand. This can create the risk of CFS, ME, fibromyalgia and autoimmune inflammatory disorders like lupus and rheumatoid arthritis, as well as complete burnout.

Symptoms of impending burnout can include:
- difficulties with concentration and memory
- brain fog
- insomnia
- low stress tolerance and irritability
- lethargy and fatigue

- light-headedness when standing up
- allergies
- PMS (premenstrual syndrome)
- more frequent coughs and colds

Of course, you can experience some or all of these symptoms, to a greater or lesser degree, for other reasons. But if you know you are pushing yourself, and you have several long-standing but minor health problems that might be related to your lifestyle, think about what you can do to avoid it escalating into a major problem with long-term consequences.

Take these vital warning signs seriously: your body is trying to tell you something.

SMALL STEPS
In times of stress, try to take a moment to check in with your body and see if you recognise any of the symptoms or warning signs identified in this chapter.

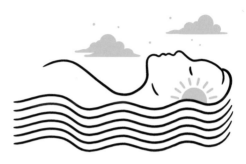

The Limbic System

The limbic system in the brain plays a significant role in regulating our emotional life and how we respond to the world. It links the thinking, feeling part of us to our physical bodies.

Here comes the science...

You may want to skip this part, but bear in mind that if you understand how your body works and what it tries to do to keep you functioning, you may then be able to both identify the warning signs of burnout and take steps to avoid it.

THE AUTONOMIC NERVOUS SYSTEM

The brain is the headquarters of all activity in the body, and its first priority is to keep the lungs breathing, the heart beating and the physical body functioning. This happens automatically via the autonomic nervous system (ANS), which combines the unique balancing act of the sympathetic nervous system (SNS) and the parasympathetic nervous system (PNS). It's the SNS that acts as an accelerator on our reactions, while the PNS acts as a brake (see page 55).

All this activity originates in the limbic system of the brain, home to the thalamus, hypothalamus, amygdala and hippocampus.

- **Thalamus:** The gateway through which all sensory information from the physical body (apart from the nose) is processed.
- **Hypothalamus:** Connected to almost every other part of the brain, this controls numerous critical functions, including hormone regulation.
- **Amygdala:** The most primitive part of the brain, its fight/flight/freeze response allows us to short-circuit the brain's cortex, privileging the survival response over rational thought when we react to actual, or perceived, threat.
- **Hippocampus:** Responsible for memory organisation and storage, this connects physical senses to emotion, for example linking certain smells to particular memories.

Although we can make the distinction with our rational minds based on previous knowledge or experience, our physical bodies don't actually distinguish between physical or psychological discomfort: both cause a similar physical reaction. So, an unkind or hurtful word really can leave us feeling wounded and evoke a similar physical reaction to a slap in the face. When we are nervous, we may talk about having the physical feeling of 'butterflies' in our stomachs or experiencing a 'sinking feeling'. We might say we feel 'gutted' by something unkind someone said. The old saying, 'Sticks and stones may break my bones, but words can never hurt me,' isn't actually true; hurt feelings really can provoke feelings of physical pain. There is even such a thing as 'broken heart syndrome': its technical name is Takotsubo cardiomyopathy, and it's often found where there's been a recent history of severe (usually negative, sometimes happy) emotional or physical stress.

This is why we can be so badly affected by what we believe other people may think or say about us, either to our faces, behind our backs or on social media, as well as the effect of our own internal critic, which relentlessly pushes us towards unrealistic goals and aims for perfection. Being aware of how strong a reaction we can have to this sort of pressure, and how it might contribute to the personal levels of stress that can lead to burnout, is important to remember when considering the impact of social and other media on your life (see page 107).

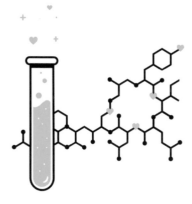

Feel-Good Hormones

Along with those stress-hormones adrenaline and cortisol, we also have feel-good hormones available to us to help balance our stress response. Knowing about these can be helpful in persuading us of the value of creating more opportunities in our lives for the activities that fire them up. Social, fun activities that activate the reward and pleasure centres in the brain can go a long way towards counteracting the stresses of life.

Endorphins

Endorphins are produced by the pituitary gland and central nervous system in response to physical stress and pain, even that caused by positive physical exercise. Similar in chemical composition to morphine, endorphins act as a natural painkiller and sedative by activating opioid receptors in the brain. When released during physical exercise, they trigger positive feelings and can create a natural 'high'. They are also produced to some extent in response to emotional stress and pain; to the body, pain is pain, and it makes little distinction between whether it's emotional or physical.

Serotonin

Serotonin is another feel-good neurotransmitter produced not only in the brain but also in the gut. It helps with the regulation of mood, sexual desire, sleep, appetite, memory and learning. A deficit in serotonin, or in the brain's ability to access it, is linked with depression. This is why a range of antidepressant drugs, called selective serotonin reuptake inhibitors, or SSRIs, were developed.

The ability to make best use of the serotonin in our bodies may also be in our genes. In 2011, behavioural economists at the London School of Economics asked more than 2,500 people how satisfied they were with their lives while also analysing their DNA for the 5-HTT gene, which is responsible for how effectively nerve cells manage to distribute serotonin. The study compared the subject's genetic type with their answer to the question, 'How satisfied are you with your life as a whole?', to which they could give one of five possible answers: very satisfied, satisfied, dissatisfied, very dissatisfied or neither.

"Of course, our well-being isn't determined by this one gene – other genes and especially experience throughout the course of life will continue to explain the majority of variations in individual happiness. But this finding helps to explain why we each have a unique baseline level of happiness and why some people tend to be naturally happier than others, and that's in no small part due to our individual genetic make-up."

JAN-EMMANUEL DE NEVE, lse.ac.uk

Dopamine

Dopamine activates the pleasure centre of the brain. We produce it in anticipation of rewards and it motivates us towards doing something that results in a pleasurable outcome. It's also the hormone generated when we 'fall in love', when our pleasure centre is highly activated. This motivates our actions towards the focus of our feelings. The downside is that the brain finds dopamine highly addictive, so it also lies at the heart of addiction, whether to love or slot machines.

Oxytocin

This hormone promotes positive, optimistic feelings, builds self-esteem and trust and is really easy to produce. All you have to do is hug someone! Even thinking positively about someone or something can do it. Oxytocin release also occurs between mother and baby during breastfeeding to promote bonding, as well as during sexual intimacy and orgasm, leading to feelings of security and closeness and earning it the nickname 'the love hormone'. It's also what makes us able to empathise, trust and love one another, so the more we do to create it and spread it around, the more content we could be.

SMALL STEPS

A hug from someone you love can give you a boost of oxytocin and release feelings of positivity.

"My bounty is as boundless as the sea, My love as deep. The more I give to thee, The more I have, for both are infinite."

WILLIAM SHAKESPEARE, *Romeo and Juliet*

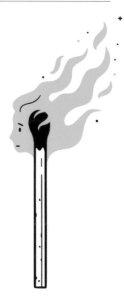

Inflammation

Recent research has drawn attention to the role inflammation can have on our neurophysiology, and those neurological processes that may increase our tendency towards those symptoms of anxiety and depression that are so often features of burnout. At this point it's not clear what comes first: the stress that causes the anxiety, or the anxiety that aggravates the stress response. Suffice to say that anything we can consciously do to reduce this stress cycle can help us to avoid or recover from burnout and protect our neurological health.

While inflammation is part of the body's normal immune response, it also occurs in response to stress whether this is physical or emotional.

The stress hormones we secrete in response to emotional stress are the same as those secreted in response to a threat to our physical survival. Physical threats to the body include actual infection, wound trauma or damage, not just the anticipation of them.Stress hormones like cortisol and adrenaline are, by nature, pro-inflammatory, because inflammation at the site of physical trauma is the first part of an immune response. Remember, our bodies don't make much distinction between physical and emotional trauma, so this inflammatory response can take place in reaction to an emotional event too, because of the stress hormones released.

Exercise

Regular moderate, low-intensity exercise, like walking, yoga, Pilates or swimming can help to 'mop up' excess stress hormones. Avoid high-intensity exercise if you are trying to avoid or recover from burnout; while it can give you an endorphin 'high' (see page 35), this is in direct response to the stress caused to the body, which will also release pro-inflammatory stress hormones cortisol and adrenaline. High-intensity exercise when you are trying to avoid or recover from burnout is unhelpful, as it just reinforces your body and mind's sense that you are under threat.

Our sedentary lifestyles can also contribute to inflammation and there is some evidence that regular light-to-moderate exercise goes some way towards preventing this. Certainly, there is a direct link between a sedentary lifestyle and risk factors for obesity, diabetes, cardiovascular disease and generally shortened life expectancy: all good reasons to stay active.

SMALL STEPS

You don't have to run a marathon or join a kick-boxing class. Try a gentle walk with a friend or a chilled-out morning swim.

Foods that help

All the foods that we consider to be 'healthy' – often plant based, unprocessed, and freshly sourced, cooked and eaten – should be placed high on any list to support our bodies if we are trying to avoid or recover from burnout. Some foods contain substances that are actively anti-inflammatory (listed below). Pro-inflammatory foods, however, include simple, high-glycaemic (GI) carbohydrates (see page 77) and dairy products, so opt instead for complex (low-GI) carbs and milk substitutes like oat milk, itself a complex carb, or almond milk, which contains magnesium instead. Use polyunsaturated fats like virgin olive oil rather than saturated fats for cooking. Walnut oil also contains anti-inflammatory omega-3 fatty acids.

BALANCE CARBS WITH PROTEINS

Always opt for low-GI, complex carbs, but balance these with protein when you eat, to help control insulin release and prevent the wildly fluctuating blood sugar spikes that can occur when eating simple, high-GI carbs alone.

ANTIOXIDANTS

Oxidation is a by-product of normal cell metabolism, and it creates something called 'free radicals', which are part of the body's immune response. If there is an imbalance between these and antioxidants, however, free radicals can be a cause of oxidative stress, which can cause inflammation. Eating a diet that's high in antioxidants can help, especially when we are trying to improve our health or when we are in recovery from any form of stress.

Anti-inflammatory foods

- **Garlic:** Contains diallyl disulphide, which limits the effect of pro-inflammatory cytokines (small protein molecules that trigger the body's inflammatory response).
- **Ginger:** Contains gingerol, which is a powerful anti-inflammatory antioxidant.
- **Carrots and sweet potatoes:** Contain beta-carotene, an antioxidant that is also converted by the body into vitamin A, which supports the immune system.
- **Tomatoes:** Contain high quantities of anti-inflammatory antioxidant lycopene. Cooking tomatoes in olive oil actually increases their lycopene content.
- **Red (bell) peppers:** Contain the antioxidant quercetin, which is also found in onions and apples.
- **Olive oil, particularly extra-virgin:** Contains oleocanthal, an antioxidant.
- **Berries, particularly blueberries:** Contain anti-inflammatory anthocyanins, along with fibre and vitamins.
- **Grapes:** Contain resveratrol (also found in red wine) a type of antioxidant.

- **Dark chocolate:** This needs to be at least 70 per cent cacao, which isn't to everyone's taste. It contains flavanols, which are anti-inflammatory antioxidants.
- **Mushrooms:** Contain B vitamins and antioxidants.
- **Walnuts:** Contain polyphenols as well as omega-3 fatty acids, which help reduce pro-inflammatory cytokines.
- **Turmeric:** Contains curcumin, a powerful anti-inflammatory antioxidant.
- **Fatty fish:** Contain anti-inflammatory omega-3 fatty acids eicosapentaenoic acid (EPA) and docosahexaenoic acid (DHA).
- **Broccoli, kale and cauliflower:** Broccoli in particular is rich in the antioxidant sulphoraphane.
- **Avocados:** Contain monounsaturated fat, magnesium and fibre.
- **Green tea:** Contains high quantities of epigallocatechin-3-gallate (EGCG), which reduces the production of pro-inflammatory cytokines.

SMALL CHANGES
Try swapping your morning coffee for a cup of green tea.

Supplements

When it comes to supplements, bear in mind that these should supplement a good diet rather than compensate for a poor one. Always aim to ensure that the foods you eat provide good nutrients and only supplement when necessary, perhaps if you are vegan and want to ensure an adequate vitamin B intake.

The one supplement that has a proven anti-inflammatory effect (see page 154) and which may be difficult to increase through diet alone, is Omega-3 essential fatty acids EPA (eicosapentaenoic acid) and DHA (docosahexaenoic acid). If you do choose to take an omega-3 supplement, make sure you select one is pharmaceutical grade and provides a daily dose of around 1000mg of active ingredient (not 1000mg of 'fish oil' that may only have a small quantity of EFAs). Do not, however, increase your intake of Omega-6 EFAs, which can be pro-inflammatory in excess, and which already exist in high concentration in many people's diets, from vegetable oils like sunflower and rapeseed, cereal-fed animal fats and are also an ingredient in many processed foods.

SIGNS AND SYMPTOMS: RECAP

- Pay attention to the warning signs of burnout, such as emotional, physical and mental exhaustion and a sense of being cut off and ineffective.
- Subjecting ourselves to relentless stress means our bodies are unable to return to a healthy 'baseline' state.
- Our bodies' response to emotional and physical trauma is similar, so we can still have an inflammatory response to emotional stress.
- Feel-good hormones like endorphins and serotonin can help balance the stress response.
- Gentle exercise and anti-inflammatory foods can help ease inflammation.

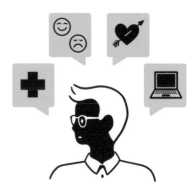

Quiz: How Close Are You to Burnout?

This quiz covers four key areas of life: work, health, mood and relationships.

Everyone's circumstances are different, and we all have different levels of resilience. You may already know that things feel a bit wobbly, but this more objective assessment can be quite revealing about the steps you may need to take now to avoid complete burnout.

Complete the quiz without thinking too much about the answers, just responding to which of the three options most accurately sums up your situation. The idea is to get a quick overview of how you *feel* about things, and your perception of your personal situation. Often, quite simple measures can correct an imbalance and change a situation that's causing you stress.

It is also useful is to look at the balance between these four key areas, because they all have an effect, both singularly and combined. It may be that in one or two areas, all is fine, but in others there are problems. Being mindful of the impact of one area on another can help you to avoid an escalation of problems, and work out the steps you might need to take, right now, to redress the balance.

HEALTH

Do you often wake up feeling as tired as when you went to sleep?

A. Never.

B. Sometimes.

C. Always.

Does it take you longer than 20 minutes to fall asleep?

A. No.

B. Only when I'm stressed.

C. It regularly takes me an hour at least to drop off.

Do you wake before the alarm goes off?

A. No.

B. Sometimes, if I've slept badly.

C. I usually wake up long before the alarm goes off.

Do you eat regular meals and enjoy your food?

A. Yes.

B. I often find I'm snacking to save time.

C. I have to watch what I eat because of my allergies.

Do you enjoy preparing the food you eat?

A. Yes.

B. I enjoy it when I have time.

C. I don't have time to cook and rely on fast food and takeaways.

How often do you exercise?

A. Two or three times a week.

B. I try to do something at least once a week.

C. My only exercise is walking to the bus stop.

How many days off sick for minor ailments have you had in the last year?

A. A few – no more than a week.

B. Several weeks.

C. I'm off sick at least once a month.

MOOD

Do you ever find yourself irritable and snappy for no obvious reason?

A. Seldom.

B. Sometimes.

C. Often.

Do you feel negatively affected by current news events?

A. No, unless they're personal to me.

B. Only on a bad day.

C. Yes, it can affect my whole day.

Do you tend to worry about things you can't change?

A. No.

B. They sometimes concern me.

C. Yes

RELATIONSHIPS

How supported do you feel by your colleagues at work?

A. Very; they're a good bunch.

B. Some days are better than others.

C. I feel that I am constantly being undermined.

How much time do you spend with your family?

A. A lot. I like hanging out with them.

B. We meet for family occasions but seldom in between.

C. I hardly ever speak to them.

Do you feel you spend enough time with those special to you?

A. Generally, yes.

B. Less than I'd like.

C. There's no one special.

WORK

Do you look forward to going to work?

A. Yes, it energises me.

B. Most days it's O.K.

C. I often dread it.

Do you feel that the job you do is within your capability?

A. Yes, pretty much.

B. Sometimes I feel a little stretched.

C. I constantly fear being caught out.

Do you find your work challenging but rewarding?

A. Yes.

B. Sometimes.

C. Never.

After work, do you enjoy relaxing and socialising?

A. Mostly.

B. When I can.

C. I'm usually too exhausted.

YOUR RESULTS

Mostly As

You appear to have a good balance and there's not much reason to worry. It is important to regularly reassess the balance between different areas of life and take action if any one of these becomes problematic.

Mostly Bs

Generally, dealing with stress in one area will help you to rebalance how you are managing overall. It's good to be aware, however, that if the balance shifts so that more than two areas are stressful at the same time, it's likely to become a problem.

Mostly Cs

The warning signs are all there and the culmination of their effects over time could easily lead to burnout. If this feels problematic, take steps immediately and factor in some serious reassessment, in order to create a better balance in all aspects of your life.

02

·

Be Stress
Smart

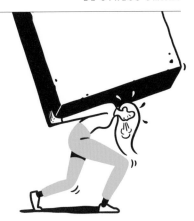

What is Stress?

Our ability to respond to stress isn't in itself a problem, but it becomes one when high levels of stress become habitual and overwhelming, whether because the stress is extreme or because it has gone on for too long. A continual stress response in the body creates constantly higher levels of stress hormones adrenaline and cortisol. Functioning at a perpetual level of red alert is detrimental to both our psychological and physical health.

According to the UK's Health and Safety Executive (HSE), stress, depression or anxiety accounted for 57 per cent of all 'sick days' in 2017/2018. Comparable rates occur all around the world and as a result greater acknowledgement is now being given to the impact of mental health on productivity.

Our stress response is regulated by our autonomic nervous system (ANS). There are two parts to the ANS, the sympathetic nervous system (SNS) and the parasympathetic nervous system (PNS). The SNS acts as an accelerator, the PNS as a brake, and they work together to balance our response.

Stress activates the SNS. When we respond to emergencies or react to danger, the SNS triggers the hormones that make the heart beat faster; our blood pressure rises, our breathing rate increases, and our muscles mobilise for the fight/flight/freeze response. This response is essential to our survival if we are faced with a physical threat: for example, if we inadvertently step into the street and a fast-approaching car sounds its horn.

In turn, the PNS acts as a brake on the SNS, slowing down our heart rate, relaxing the body, and generally calming everything down to allow the body's systems to return to normal. The PNS is controlled by the vagus nerve, a cranial nerve that connects the brain to the body and which starts at the base of the skull and travels down through the nervous system, past the throat, heart, diaphragm and gut. Its function is to calm all those body systems as required, producing an optimal state for all the other systems to function.

What can we do?

First, learn to recognise the particular symptoms of your own stress. We are all individual in our responses and some of us are more susceptible to stress than others. But being aware, and mindful, of our personal stress response helps us take the steps we need to rebalance.

What are your personal stress responses?
◆ Pounding heart? ◆ Distracted thoughts? ◆ 'Wired' feeling?

Now try to identify your tipping point: the stage where you go from coping with the stress in your life to not coping with it. Being aware of this is helpful in identifying strategies to manage stress and how you react to it.

Rumination

One of the side effects of stress, and one that leads to further stress, is the habit of rumination. Replaying the memory of a stressful experience over and over can activate similar pathways in the brain to those that were activated by the original experience. Just thinking about it can keep the stress reaction to the original occurrence 'switched on' long after the event and can cause the experience to be perceived as more distressing than it actually was.

FIRST AID

At the first sign of stress, whether this is in response to missing the bus, having to make a difficult phone call or receiving bad news, it's good to avoid any escalation of the stress response *immediately* by taking some steadying breaths (see page 60) to activate the PNS, applying that brake to the SNS. Deep, slow belly breathing that makes the chest cavity expand and the diaphragm contract activates the vagus nerve, and this will trigger a relaxation rather than a stress response. Through this simple measure, your calm breathing tells your body that all is well, and the mind follows.

Regular practice

You don't need to wait until you've had a fright to learn breathing techniques (see page 60). Regular practice of these techniques will make them more accessible when you need them. Breathing techniques are associated with many exercise routines that link body and mind, for example yoga, T'ai Chi and Pilates. Breathing techniques are used to slow, steady and relax the body, which not only helps to relieve muscle tension, but also to calm the mind.

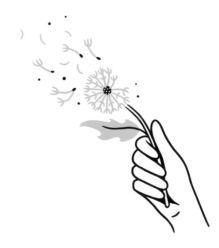

Breathe

There is a direct link between the body and mind that we can tap into through controlling our breath, and we can use this connection to put a brake on our stress response.

Many of us breathe poorly most of the time, mostly out of habit. We tend to take three or four breaths using only the upper part of our lung capacity. This form of shallow breathing is very tiring, not only because we expend unnecessary energy, but also because it reduces our oxygen intake per breath. When we are under stress, this shallow breathing causes us to over-breathe, which leads to hyperventilation.

Once we are breathing like this, our brain receives a message that the body is anxious, which can trigger the stress response.

We breathe shallowly when in fight/flight/freeze mode, in response to the secretion of stress hormones. Because of this, when we breathe shallowly out of habit, it makes us more stressed than we might otherwise feel. Deliberately breathing more calmly will de-stress us, because the very act of consciously doing so sends a message from the body to the brain that everything is now O.K., the emergency is over, and it can stop pumping out all the unnecessary adrenaline and cortisol that is over-stimulating us and revving us up.

Shallow breathing also alters the balance of oxygen and carbon dioxide in the blood, making it more acidic, and over time our muscles feel chronically tired and weakened from this effect. Tired muscles overcompensate by tensing up, increasing physical tension overall, which in turn makes us feel emotionally tense and stressed.

Poor breathing patterns can become a habit, and begin to feel normal, as can the feelings of stress that this provokes. It sets up a vicious circle, and one that affects us both physically and emotionally. But the great news is that one simple change — how you breathe — can make a huge difference to how you feel. And this can be consciously practiced and learned.

Calm breathing exercise
- Lie comfortably on the floor, with your knees bent and feet flat on the floor or sit upright in a chair, legs uncrossed, with your feet flat on the floor.

- Consciously relax your neck and shoulders. Let your arms rest by your sides with your palms turned upwards.
- Breathe gently through your nose and into your belly until you see it gently rise, for a slow count of five.
- Pause and hold that breath for a count of five, then gently exhale through your mouth for another slow count of five.
- While doing this, try to clear your mind of all other thoughts or, if this is difficult, close your eyes and visualise a pebble dropping into a pool of water and gently sinking, slowly, down.
- Repeat this breathing cycle 10 times, then see how your regular breathing adjusts.

You can use this practice of calm breathing at any time you feel tense or stressed, or as the basis of any meditation practice. The more you use this technique, the more easily you will be able to access its calming effect when you need it.

SMALL CHANGES

Try setting your alarm ten minutes earlier in the morning to give you time to practise this simple breathing technique. It only takes a few minutes and can make a huge difference.

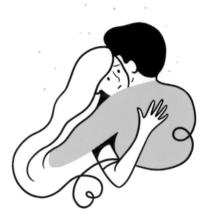

Connect

We are wired for connection; it's an important physiological need in humans. Humans are, by nature, social beings, and close connections not only help our positive emotions to thrive, they also help protect us against the harmful effects of stress.

Physical touch can also help to anchor us. A hug from someone we love helps release the hormone oxytocin (see page 36) which provides a feeling of natural calm by decreasing cortisol and adrenaline and lowering blood pressure. Even just thinking loving and positive thoughts about someone you cherish works.

However stressful some of our relationships may be, social isolation is more damaging. Loneliness is very stressful. We can feel lonely even when we're in a relationship or surrounded by people. Equally, we might enjoy solitude, but not like feeling isolated. Social isolation can increase anxiety, depression and other mental health problems, and can become a feature of burnout. We may feel as if everyone is shunning us (and our use of social media and checking for 'likes' can exacerbate this). But often the truth is that it's our own reluctance to test the waters of human exchange that is keeping us isolated.

If life has got so busy or out of kilter that we no longer have time to foster positive relationships at work, at home or at play, this needs to be addressed. Try just getting into the habit of acknowledging neighbours, responding to the person serving you, making eye contact, smiling when it's appropriate and exchanging small talk. There's a reason we talk about the weather: it's there, it's impersonal and it allows us to take the temperature of any casual exchange. Join a sports team or a book club, source local communities where you can make new connections and cherish your old ones. Friendships and existing relationships need nurturing. It's always a two-way process and burnout can see us neglecting those real-time social connections that can nourish us.

SMALL CHANGES
Take a moment to smile and properly acknowledge the barista when you get your coffee, or the cashier when you're doing your shopping. A small moment of human connection will benefit you both.

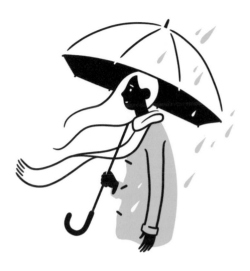

Increasing Resilience

Resilience describes our ability to bounce back from bad experiences and tough situations; an ability to recover quickly from difficulties or setbacks in a positive way. It has become something of a buzz word, especially when people talk about the 'snowflake' generation needing more resilience. The good news, however, is that resilience is something that we can consciously foster and develop at any age.

"Recovery [from burnout] is that point at which resilience makes a serious contribution. The capacity to recover from the physical, mental, or emotional demands of the job matters. Some recovery occurs at work, but the large part of recovery occurs away from work while resting, having fun and sleeping. The capacity to recover more thoroughly or more readily makes a difference when tackling a challenging work life."

PROFESSOR MICHAEL LEITER, Organisational Psychologist

One of the key features of resilience is feeling that we have some influence over events in our lives. We can't always predict or control what life throws at us, but we always have a choice in how we respond. Focusing on what we can do is far more helpful, than adopting a victim mentality and asking, 'Why me?'. There's no need to blame others or feel helpless when we see challenge in adversity.

Developing resilience to life's adversities can be learned at any age, and these skills are often developed in response to managing and overcoming difficulties in childhood. In fact, a childhood without challenges and adversities can make resilience in adulthood less immediately possible. However, resilience is made more attainable at any age by an environment of loving support.

Break it down

Rather than feel overwhelmed by a setback, try to keep a sense of perspective and see it in context. It's not the end of the world; it's just something that's happened, and from which you can move on. There may even be useful lessons to learn from the situation. Ask for feedback from a trusted friend, mentor or coach, too: sometimes our subjective view of a situation is inaccurate and an objective take on events can help us gain useful perspective.

Avoid catastrophising

'We won't make a drama out of a crisis' was a well-known 1980s advertising slogan in the UK (thank you, Commercial Union), and there's something to be said for reminding ourselves of this phrase when confronting a dilemma or stressful situation. It may feel as though something awful has happened to you, but try to examine what you *know* about what's actually happened and think of an alternative or more positive outcome from there. Focus on this rather than mulling over how awful you feel. And don't waste time worrying about what might happen in the future. Imagining the worst is futile and just saps energy that could be put to better use.

SMALL CHANGES

Next time a situation makes you feel upset or stressed, ask someone you trust for their feedback on it. An objective point of view can help you see things differently.

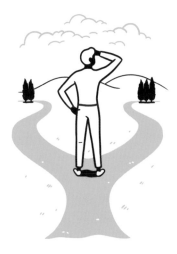

Managing Uncertainty

Uncertainty is a fact of life. It is also a potential stressor that can erode our sense of agency over our own lives. Learning to manage uncertainty can be helpful in terms of preventing the sort of low-level stress that can contribute to burnout.

As an unconscious strategy, we often attempt to solve uncertainties in our own lives in an effort to manage our anxiety about situations outside our control, from climate emergencies to political elections. However, trying to solve uncertainties, big or small, can also lead to rumination (see page 57) and the sort of worrying that just makes us feel more stressed. When we are trying to avoid or recover from burnout, it's important to be mindful about worrying about things we can't control.

"It is impossible to control outcomes or results, although most of us have been programmed from a very young age to believe otherwise. The idea that we can perform actual 'magic' causes tremendous dysfunction, unnecessary suffering and prevents the development of emotional resilience."

CHRISTOPHER DINES, Author of *Mindfulness Burnout Prevention*

We may find ourselves asking perpetual questions about the future, often based on information we don't have or can't know, and constantly ruminating on these. Is this the right job for me? Am I doing the right thing? Will I regret doing this or not doing that (whatever this or that might be)? This constant attempt to manage uncertainty can become exhausting and immobilising.

The trick is to recognise that uncertainties actually exist and check back on the reality of the situation. When we feel uncertain, it's an opportunity to be curious and open-minded. We need to accept that sometimes we just don't, can't or won't know what the answer is right now (or perhaps ever), but we can trust that it will probably be O.K.

This doesn't mean we are powerless in the face of uncertainty. There are steps we can take that can be very helpful.

- Instead of imagining what might go wrong, consciously visualise how well things might go.
- Keep going. There's much to recommend just putting one foot in front of the other and doing what you can.
- If you feel powerless about the state of the world, join a community movement or political party. Make sure you recycle, try to buy less: be the change you want to see in the world.
- Look at what is within your control: how you treat yourself and others, for example.
- Accept that uncertainty is a part of life and learn to see it more positively, as something that opens up opportunities to be embraced.

Another way to manage uncertainty is to recognise those areas where you are already successfully doing so. Every day, you already do hundreds of things without concern, whether it's crossing the road or eating in the canteen, because the probability of being run over or getting food poisoning is low, as you know from past experience. Applying some rational logic when you are calm is one way to reduce the worry voice in your head.

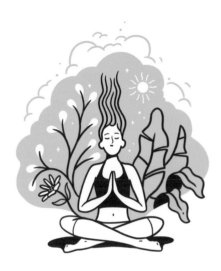

Living Mindfully

Mindfulness is often recommended when we are stressed, but it is much easier to utilise in moments of need if we practice it regularly. It's an extremely useful tool to help calm a stressed mind, and also helps reduce rumination (see page 57) because it's a way of letting those recurring and cyclic thoughts go.

DAILY MINDFULNESS MEDITATION

- ◆ Turn off any devices or notifications that might disturb you.
- ◆ Set yourself a timer. Just five or ten minutes to begin with is fine.
- ◆ Find a sitting position that's comfortable for you and notice your body adjusting into it.
- ◆ Focus on your breath and consciously feel the sensation of gently breathing through your nose into your belly.
- ◆ Notice when your mind wanders and return your focus to your breathing.
- ◆ Don't engage with your thoughts: just allow them to drift past without conscious judgement.
- ◆ Keep returning your focus to your breathing until the timer sounds.

Use this mindfulness meditation practice regularly and whenever you feel the need to calm your mind and relax your body.

"Mindfulness (present-moment awareness) is deliberately focusing our attention on our thoughts, emotions, feelings, sensations and mental activity without losing awareness of what is happening in the present moment. It is essentially being in a state of present-moment awareness and maintaining clarity without being swayed or distracted by mental commentary."

CHRISTOPHER DINES, Author of *Mindfulness Burnout Prevention*

You can also help yourself by trying to be mindful throughout your day, every day.

- Do one thing at a time, rather than multitask; multitasking is the antithesis of mindfulness.
- Try not to stand in judgement of yourself or others: acknowledge your thoughts and let them go.
- Respond rather than react. Take five mindful breaths if you need to give yourself a moment, then respond.
- Be aware that how you feel physically – tired, hungry, dehydrated, ill or in pain– can make the body more stressed, which may hinder feelings of calm.
- At least once a day, acknowledge three good things in your life and give thanks for their presence.

> "When we are reactive, falling victim to our immediate thoughts or emotions, we are not always acting in our own self-interest. Mindfulness provides a great tool for developing more self-acceptance, which helps us build our compassion for others."

LISA FIRESTONE PHD, Clinical Psychologist

Rewiring the brain

Although we can't literally rewire our brain, it's a useful metaphor because changing the way we think can actually change the way the brain works by creating new neurological pathways that make different connections. When we worry and ruminate on negative thoughts, our thoughts run along well-worn neurological pathways, to which we return with ease, their familiarity providing some sort of 'known' comfort. Mindfulness can help alter these pathways by not reinforcing negative thought patterns. This is what lies at the heart of cognitive behavioural therapy (CBT, see page 83). By consciously changing what we think about and how we think about it, we can literally change the way the brain works by creating new neurological pathways and connections.

Exercise (see page 159), not least because it helps in the production of brain-derived neurotrophic factor (BDNF, see page 161) can also help to support the creation of new neurological connections. Exercising mindfully might just be the best thing you can do for yourself when rewiring your brain.

Natural benefits

Biophilia, a love of and response to the natural world, has a very profound, positive effect on mood. Nature, and spending time in natural surroundings, is restorative and something which we should factor into a daily mindfulness practice to help relieve the stress that can contribute to burnout. Researchers from Stanford University (see page 160) found that spending time outdoors had a soothing effect the brain. It's also beneficial when we can to exercise (see page 159) outdoors rather than in a gym or studio, combining the benefits of both.

Wherever and whenever possible take some time out, outside. Notice the sensations of the air, sometimes soft and warm, sometimes rough or cold. Listen to the sounds of the leaves stirring on the trees, or underfoot as the seasons change. Notice the birdsong, or the sound of water tumbling. See the clouds shift and the light change. Notice how a well-known view on a walk can change through the day or time of year. Finding opportunities to mindfully notice, observe and reflect on the natural beauty that we can see, hear, smell and feel around us is very grounding and restorative and will support us in avoiding or recovering from burnout.

Gardening, too, combines gentle physical labour with concentrating on a task that will eventually reap its own reward. If there's no garden or allotment available, bringing the natural world into the home with beautiful plants or window boxes creates similar opportunities and culinary herbs can even be grown to use when cooking. Working with the soil, weeding, sowing or planting is very grounding. It helps us focus on the present moment while also looking towards a positive future in anticipation of the growth, blossoming or fruition of our efforts. In growing plants, we have to care for and nurture something and this also reminds us of the importance of nurturing and caring for ourselves.

SMALL CHANGES

Set aside five or ten minutes a day to practice the mindfulness meditation on page 76.

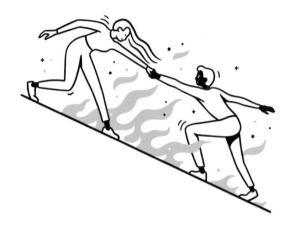

When to Ask for Help

Sometimes, however hard we try, we can't manage to unravel the circumstances that can lead to burnout on our own. Things may have escalated to the point where our physical and emotional health has become so out of kilter that we need help to get back on track. Sometimes, too, it's very hard to recognise when we are close to, or hitting, burnout, and the first recognition of this may come from family, friends or work colleagues who have noticed our struggle. There is no shame in acknowledging that things have become tricky and asking for the help that could in fact mean that complete burnout and longer term problems can be prevented.

Talk to someone

Different approaches work for different people. Taking the first step of telling a close friend that you are struggling may set you on the path towards avoiding, or recovering from, burnout. It's not always easy to find the words to express how we're feeling, and this can be further complicated by not wishing to burden others.

Sometimes just putting in place the strategies outlined in this book, and allowing the time necessary for these to work, can be enough (although you should bear in mind that it's unlikely to be a quick fix). But if part of the problem is, for example, a physical health issue or your work environment, this needs to be specifically addressed. If you believe your burnout is related to your workplace, find out if your employer has a mental health strategy in place, either through the Human Resources (HR) team or occupational health department. There may also be a trained mental health first aider among your colleagues.

Talking treatments

Alongside the steps you need to take for your physical health, a doctor or physician may be able to advise you on what talking treatments might be suitable, and what may be available to you in your area. In many cases, once you have an idea of what might be most helpful, you can self-refer. Whatever you decide, it's worth considering a) what you would like it to achieve, and b) the approach and training of any therapist you work with. It's also important that any therapist consulted is properly trained and supervised and abides by an acceptable standard of professional ethics. Most are accredited to a professional body: in the UK, for example, the British Association for Counselling and Psychotherapy is a professional body representing those registered with them and to which therapists are accountable.

COGNITIVE BEHAVIOURAL THERAPY (CBT)

This helps you to identify and change those negative thoughts that contribute to your feeling anxious and depressed. For mild depression, computerised CBT might be offered, either for use alone or in addition to sessions with a CBT-trained therapist.

MINDFULNESS-BASED COGNITIVE THERAPY (MBCT)

This approach focuses on being mindful, by consistently paying attention to the present moment and viewing life in a non-judgmental way, rather than persistently ruminating on worries. In addition, MBCT can form the basis of group therapy.

COUNSELLING

This involves talking with someone who is trained to listen with empathy and acceptance. It allows you to express your feelings and helps you to find your own solutions to your problems through a structured relationship, and feedback from, your therapist.

PSYCHOTHERAPY

With a focus on your past experiences and how these may be contributing to your experiences and feelings in the present, psychotherapy can be short or long-term. In addition, it may be more frequent and intensive than counselling, and may delve deeply into your childhood and significant relationships.

GROUP THERAPY

Run by a trained therapist, this allows a group of people to work together and support each other with their problems. Some people find it easier to talk with others who have had similar experiences and find their shared insights helpful.

EMDR

If by any chance the cause of burnout is an unresolved case of post-traumatic stress disorder (PTSD) finding a therapist who is also trained in eye movement desensitisation reprogramming (EMDR) can be extremely beneficial. The UK's National Institute of Clinical Excellence recommends its use to help those for whom traumatic memories trigger the stress response.

Medication

In some cases, either in the short term or in the long term, medication can be very helpful for anxiety or depression associated with burnout. It can sometimes be helpful in resolving initial symptoms while addressing some of the underlying causes, and selective serotonin reuptake inhibitors (SSRIs) are sometimes prescribed for this purpose. These are usually well tolerated, but for many people it takes up to four weeks for them to have an actual effect while adjusting to some of the common side effects: it depends on the individual.

Self-help

Whatever the cause of any unhappiness, depression or other mental health issues that may contribute to or be caused by burnout, the self-help measures outlined in this book should also be used. Whatever your situation, paying attention to your physical health and well-being will support your mental health. Good nutrition, regular exercise, adequate downtime and good sleep habits are important for everyone in order to avoid or recover from burnout.

BE STRESS SMART: RECAP

- Functioning at a perpetual level of red alert is detrimental to both our psychological and physical health.
- Habitual shallow breathing creates a stress response in the body. Learning to breathe deeply (see page 60) enables us to calm and manage this reaction.
- Learn to increase your resilience to improve your ability to cope with and recover from stress.
- Learn to accept what you can and can't control.
- Adopt a practice of mindfulness.
- Ask for help.

03

·

Workplace Stress

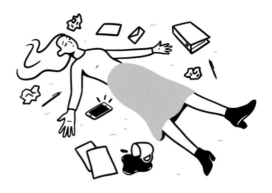

Your Workplace

If we spend just eight hours a day doing work we love in a relaxed, productive, congenial atmosphere, with friendly and supportive colleagues, we are unlikely to get burnout.

If, however, we are wrestling with long days (or nights), zero-hours contracts, a lack of job security, a difficult working environment and hostile colleagues, it can feel hard – if not impossible – to find a way to nourish ourselves well enough to deliver at work.

It is worth aiming for more balance and ease in our working life in order to be able to live happily and well.

Workplace stress is a serious issue and it tends to affect those who feel they have no control over their working day, including its hours or conditions. One downside of the gig economy is that its security is usually based on working without any safety net of sickness or holiday benefit, and this can contribute to stress.

Health legislation in many countries is quite clear about what workplace-related stress might look like. Some areas of concern are covered opposite and can provide a useful checklist. But if you are struggling, it may be worth checking legislation, and also consulting any HR or occupational health service colleagues within your organisation to ask them what kind of mental health provisions the company has in place.

Breaking down what pressure points exist for you can be a helpful first step. The demands of the job should be realistic. Is the amount of work you're being asked to do reasonable? Are you struggling to fulfil your workload in the time allotted? Do you need extra training or support to fulfil your role, and if so do you feel able to raise this with your line manager? Issues like these can seem tricky to address, especially if you are highly conscientious and want to make a good impression, or if there is an atmosphere of fear that makes speaking up difficult. However, a good employer knows how badly productivity can be affected if their workforce isn't managing or needs greater support, so it's absolutely in their interest – as well as yours – that employees aren't struggling.

THINGS TO CONSIDER

- What kind of support do you get from managers and colleagues? Sickness absence is often a good indicator of employees feeling unable to talk to their line managers or colleagues about the problems they're experiencing.

- What are your work relationships like? If these are poor, problems easily arise – especially if there are any unaddressed issues around, or inappropriate behaviour.

- How does your role fit within the organisation? Understanding what is expected of you in terms of the overall objectives of the organisation is essential.

- Has there been change at work, and if so, how is it managed? Any change within an organisation can create uncertainty and insecurity, especially if it is not well-managed.

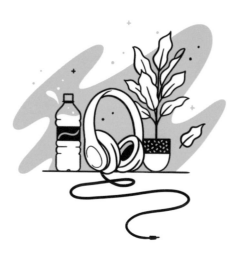

Environment

We may not have much control over our place of work, whether this is a desk space, a classroom, a shop floor or the cab of a lorry. Here are some factors to consider when you are assessing your work environment.

- Our physical environment should be well-lit and well-ventilated, with a comfortable working temperature of around 16° C (60° F) minimum and 24°C (75°F) maximum.
- There are some arguments for having our surroundings painted a relaxing pale blue, green or pink, with either plants or posters of natural environments as part of the décor.
- Noise should be within an acceptable range and shouldn't exceed 80 decibels.
- Noise nuisances – other colleagues, piped music, etc. – can also be stressful, and this should be recognised.

We may not be able to do much about the issues listed above, beyond drawing them to the attention of our line managers (if we feel able to do so). What we can learn to manage, however, are the small ways in which we can make the environment more comfortable.

- We may not be able to control the noise levels around us, but noise-cancelling headphones might help.
- Regular short breaks can help alleviate stress at work. Just getting up and walking around the office to deliver a message to a colleague rather than emailing can make a difference.
- Doing some simple chair-based or standing stretches at regular intervals can help with the physical stress of sedentary work, particularly where it involves long hours spent at computers.
- Risk factors for repetitive strain injury should be assessed by HR, and steps taken to avoid this common complaint.
- Taking a proper lunch break away from our desks, whether we go to the canteen or take a brisk walk around the block, is important, as are good hydration and regular meals (see page 151).

SMALL CHANGES

Take your lunch break: it's there for a reason. Step away from your desk, get some fresh air and eat a decent meal. You'll return feeling refreshed and have a more productive afternoon as a result.

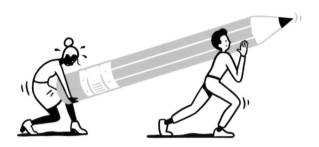

Colleagues

If we're lucky in the workplace, we'll have like-minded colleagues who are just as industrious, happy and positive as we are (on a good day)! In real life, however, nobody has perfect colleagues all the time. Managing workplace relationships takes time and emotional intelligence, and some days are more manageable than others, depending on our own feelings and mood.

Recognising and dealing with difficult people

Behavioural scientist Dr Robert Bramson identified seven key personality types who create stress for those around them. Identifying the style of our tormentors can help us find coping strategies to reduce the stress they cause us.

- **Know-it-all experts:** These can be divided into two types: those who might actually know what they are talking about; and those who consider themselves experts on the basis of very little information, but present it with such authority that it's difficult not to feel overwhelmed by them. Respond to the facts, which can be checked, and not how you feel about the person, which helps depersonalise the situation.
- **Super-agreeables:** They come across as good-humoured and willing, but never deliver. They are exasperating because they agree to everything in an effort to be liked, but constantly let you down. Agree any work-load within a time frame and confirm briefly with colleagues by email so it's clear and well-documented.
- **Indecisive stallers:** One of the most stress-inducing types, especially if you are dependent on their decision-making in order to get your own work done. The approach for super-agreeables can work well here, too.
- **Pessimists:** No matter what you say or how you present it, they always respond negatively, and often with such conviction that it's difficult not to get hooked into their negative agenda. Depersonalise this work relationship by focusing on facts while remaining consistent in seeing challenges as opportunities.
- **Silent unresponsives:** This type purposefully use silence to negatively control situations, undermining others. It can be a

form of passive aggression or a spiteful refusal to co-operate. Again, a similar approach to super-agreeables can work here.

* **Hostile aggressives:** Basically, these are the office bullies. They aim to get their own way by being hostile and using ridicule or sarcasm. Their criticism tends to be personal and they induce stress by confusing, frustrating or even frightening you. If you feel bullied, make a note of date, time and event, and escalate any fact-based concerns to your line manager.
* **Complainers:** They indulge in constant whining while refusing to take steps to change the things they are complaining about. This can be super stressful because they suck you in while ignoring helpful suggestions and wasting your time.

It's also helpful to review our own workplace behaviours and reactions and consider how we might cause stress to those around us. None of us is infallible, but given how much time we spend at work (in the UK it averages around 48 hours per week) we owe it to each other to facilitate each other's – and our own – best use of time. Actively trying to reduce second-hand stress in the workplace helps us all work more effectively.

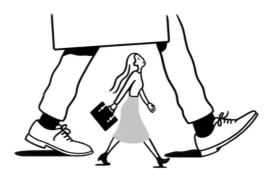

Expectations

While there are some expectations that are completely reasonable at work, for example that we will be given the respect we deserve and the resources we need to complete our tasks, it is also necessary to keep our expectations realistic. Unrealistic expectations can be very stressful and need to be addressed.

Our expectations might include:
- finding work enjoyable every day;
- managing our workload;
- working with friendly and accommodating people;
- getting promoted after a short time;
- juggling our time.

Some of these expectations might be more reasonable or realistic than others, depending on the job we do, the structure of the organisation and our position or seniority within a company. However, the bottom line is that we are usually employed to be productive members of a team. Others will often rely on us to do our jobs so that they can do theirs (and vice versa).

If, for example, you are employed as an intern, you should not expect to be running the company by the end of the first week. This is an exaggeration, of course, but sometimes our attitude can get in the way of what we can reasonably expect to achieve within a specific job description. No one who has ever become a success has done it overnight and, in most cases, it has required a lot of hard work alongside their genius! It's important to recognise not only the potential of what we do but also the limitations of our role. We should use our time to gain the skills and experience we need to progress. One of the biggest contributions any of us can make is to show up on time and do our job with good grace and as well as we can.

Stress can occur when there's a gap between our expectations of work and the reality of it. Sometimes adjusting our expectations helps; this might mean addressing issues with others, reconsidering our position, or requesting further training and support.

WORKPLACE STRESS: RECAP

- Workplace stressors, like long hours, high pressure and a poor physical and emotional environment, can all contribute to burnout.
- Think about the things that are troubling you at work and consider what options are available to you in terms of addressing them.
- Think about your colleagues and whether their behaviour is contributing towards your stress.
- Consider your expectations: how realistic are they? Having unrealistic expectations can be a cause of stress.

04

·

Social
Media Stress

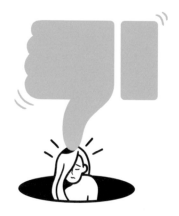

Social Media

In August 2018, research published by the UK's telecoms regulator Ofcom reported that people checked their smartphones, on average, every 12 minutes during their waking hours, with 71 per cent of respondents saying they never turn their phone off and 40 per cent saying they check their phone within five minutes of waking. It's not just emails, text or WhatsApp messages we're checking, but also social media platforms such as Twitter, Facebook and Instagram. Many of us have become victims of connectivity, never switching off, and existing in a digital bubble rather than nurturing real life connections.

This relentless digital connectivity can be very stressful, not just because of how much of our time it takes up – or, some would say, how much of our time it wastes – but also because its use can actually undermine us, sapping our self-esteem and encouraging greater isolation.

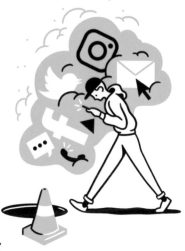

Continuous Partial Attention

Another effect of social media is that our habit of routinely switching from platform to platform to check for updates creates constant micro-interruptions, which are very stressful. Continuous partial attention (or CPA) was a phrase coined by ex-Apple and Microsoft consultant Linda Stone, who identified that we have pushed ourselves to an extreme. By adopting an always-on, anywhere, any-time, any-place behaviour, we exist in a constant state of alertness where we scan the world around us but never really give our full attention to anything. In the short term, we adapt well to these demands, but in the long term, the constantly activated stress hormones adrenaline and cortisol create a physiological hyper-alert state that constantly scans for stimuli. This provokes a sense of addiction that is temporarily assuaged by constantly checking in.

Constant, high-levels of circulating stress hormones have an inflammatory (see page 39) and detrimental effect on brain cells, suggests psychiatrist Edward Bullmore, author of *The Inflamed Mind*, who has written about the link between neuroinflammation and depression. Depression, along with anxiety, is a known factor in knocking out our ability to self-regulate our emotions. Paradoxically, the fact that we are the direct cause of this is actually good news: it means we have the potential to change our behaviour, and in so doing reclaim the brain function and cognitive health that's been disrupted and fragmented by our digitally enhanced lives.

Discontent

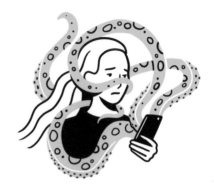

It's not just the way we use social media like Twitter, Instagram and Facebook that is problematic. It's the content of these platforms that can make social media so toxic. These mediums can also create a platform for bullying and the dissemination of fake and other distressing news. This can reinforce a negative self-view and undermine our emotional health, while also creating a sense of social isolation rather than restorative connectivity. It pays to pay attention to how we use social media, muting or unfollowing accounts the reinforce negative feedback for example, monitoring and restricting anything that can cause us psychological harm.

Young people in particular seem more at risk, with recent research showing evidence that using social media reduces time spent sleeping or exercising. Research published in the UK's *The Lancet Child & Adolescent Health* in 2019 found that those teenagers who checked social media sites more than three times a day had poorer mental health and greater psychological distress, with negative effects due to disrupted sleep, lack of exercise and cyberbullying, with a greater impact on the girls in the study. Parents were advised to ban phones from bedrooms after 10 p.m. and to encourage more physical activity.

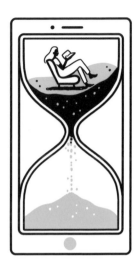

Cutting Back

There are a number of apps available for monitoring, managing or restricting our screen time, but bear in mind that using an app means you are still connected to and relying on digital devices. Deactivate accounts temporarily (or permanently) and remove apps from your smartphone, if you feel this might be helpful. Better perhaps to wean yourself off excessive digital use by trying to do something else: read a book, go to a movie (where turning off phones is requested), take a walk, eat a meal without checking your phone... basically, restore some sort of self-discipline through the benefit of alternative activities.

DIGITAL APPS TO HELP YOU CUT BACK

New apps designed to help you manage your time better come out regularly, and many of them focus on reducing the distractions offered by social media.

- **Moment:** This app tracks your smartphone usage so you can see where you're losing time.
- **Your Time on Facebook:** This is actually part of the Facebook app, and can be found under the 'Settings & Privacy' section. It will show you how much time a day you spend on the platform and gives you the option to set a daily time reminder to help reduce usage.
- **Go Cold Turkey:** This is a website blocker that won't allow you to cheat. It claims to help you 'boost your productivity and reclaim your free time by blocking distracting websites, games and applications'.
- **Stay On Task:** This app is described as a 'simple, unobtrusive way to improve your focus and get work done'. It also includes a randomly timed 'check' on progress to keep you on track.
- **AppDetox:** This is an app blocker, where you apply the blocks and take a digital detox for periods of time.
- **Space:** This app is designed to break phone addiction, with 71 per cent of users saying they reduced their smartphone usage after four weeks.

SMALL CHANGES

Try plugging in your phone to charge overnight in another room and investing in an old-school alarm clock. This could help to reduce time spent looking at social media in bed before sleeping and immediately on waking.

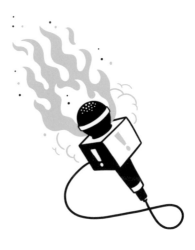

Watching the News

There are times when watching a scary movie can be fun: the anticipation of the next jump-in-your-seat moment is delicious (when we know we're in safe company, with a bag of popcorn in our hand). But this isn't true of every 'scary' thing we watch. The slow drip of negativity, harm and disaster that characterises much of what is shared via television, Twitter, gaming or gossip under the guise of entertainment or 'news' can erode positivity and undermine any sense that life is calm and ordered. Researchers from the Max Planck Institute for Human Cognitive and Brain Sciences and Dresden University of

Technology in Germany found that simply watching television could raise stress levels. The constant triggering of the limbic system (see page 29) also releases stress hormones, putting your body into a state of chronic stress, which affects all body systems.

Fake news

Fake news has become news itself and it can be hard to distinguish one from the other. Sometimes fake news is deliberately created and circulated with an agenda to deceive; and sometimes facts get misconstrued in ways that can deceive. Often fake news is linked to conspiracy theories. By and large, fake news is never good news but designed to affect us in ways that could lead to negative outcomes. All of which can be detrimental to our wellbeing. Being aware of these possibilities means being mindful of what we expose ourselves to, and what we expose others to. Social media is a powerful tool in the circulating and re-circulating of misrepresented or fake news, often items of information that a quick check can easily prove to be false, so think twice about passing it on. To protect your mental wellbeing, it's worth considering your news sources and opting for those generally accepted as most reliable. And deliberately avoid, mute or limit access if you are consciously trying to protect yourself from the worst excesses of fake news.

SOCIAL MEDIA STRESS: RECAP

- Many become addicted (see page 35) to their phones and social media. Research shows we're checking our phones every 12 minutes during waking hours.
- Our constant switching between platforms leads to Continuous Partial Attention (CPA) and increases our levels of stress hormones.
- The content on social media can leave us feeling bad about ourselves or isolated.
- The slow drip of negativity that often comes at us from these platforms and even from watching the news can trigger a stress response.
- Try to reduce your time on these platforms by using time tracking apps or enjoying different activities, like going for a walk or to the movies.

05

24-hour
Crisis Plan

Crisis Point

When the chips are down, the best resource you have is your own ability to take care of yourself. This capacity for self-care may be something you already feel you have and can rely on, or it might be something you need help from others to establish. Knowing when and how to ask for the help and support you need is an important part of taking care of yourself.

If you are approaching burnout, you need to be able to recognise the signs and take immediate steps to reduce its impact. Burnout can often happen after a long period of intense stress, whether that's work-related or not, or when something tips the balance. You may or may not have seen it coming, but, whatever your situation, you need to act now to make sure it doesn't get worse. This will allow you to navigate your own individual path from burnout to balance.

"Unless we begin with the right attitude, we will never find the right solution."

CHINESE PROVERB

Remember, you don't have to apologise for or explain the necessity of taking care of yourself. As they say on the airplane safety message, 'Please secure your own oxygen mask before assisting others with theirs'.

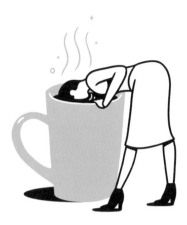

Key Signs to Watch Out For

- You are exhausted in a way that's unrelieved by sleep.

- You can't sleep even though you're overwhelmingly tired.

- You crave sugary foods and caffeine.

- Your heart is constantly pounding due to an excess of stress hormones.

- Any minor anxieties assume mammoth proportions.

- You feel hyper-emotional and tearful.

- You don't want to socialise, and life feels pointless.

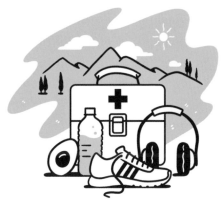

First Steps

Below are some immediate first steps that you should take if you are approaching or in burnout. It's important to recognise that these steps won't completely solve the problem – but they will start the process.

- Go through your diary and cancel any upcoming events or functions that aren't completely essential.
- Set up an 'out of office' email reply explaining that you'll be away from your desk for a while.
- Turn off your computer.
- Turn off all social media apps on your smartphone.
- Only do any exercise that is calming, such as restorative yoga, gentle walking or swimming. Don't do anything that makes your heart pound.
- Eat small amounts of nutritious and easy-to-prepare foods at regular intervals (every 3–4 hours) to maintain blood sugar equilibrium: avocados, bananas and proteins balanced with slow carbs (see page 151 for more on a restorative diet).

- Keep hydrated, but only drink water, calming tisanes or herbal teas like chamomile, roobois, lime blossom, lemon balm, mint, fennel or jasmine. Avoid caffeine.
- Take a warm (not hot) bath with lavender oil and magnesium salts.
- Wear loose, comfortable clothing and warm socks.
- Listen to calming soundscapes or music that has a rhythm slower than our heartbeat or resonates with the Alpha wave pattern in our brain. Alpha waves are on the same frequency as the Schumann Resonance, the frequency of the earth's electromagnetic field. When our brainwaves are in Alpha rhythm, we feel more grounded and in tune with the earth's energy. Bach's cello suites are a good example of Alpha wave music.
- Don't watch or listen to the news, as this can trigger a stress response. Try to disengage your thoughts for a while.
- Do some breathing exercises (see page 60) to help stimulate the vagus nerve (see page 56) and activate the deceleration effect of the parasympathetic nervous system (see page 55).
- Create a calm atmosphere in your home and sleep as much and for as long as you can.

If you can do the above for a whole day, a weekend or even a week while on holiday, you will have started the process of alleviating burnout. This is the basis on which you can move to a fuller restoration of life balance.

BURNOUT FIRST AID
These are quick and easy things you can do to ease stress and relieve immediate symptoms of burnout.

- Deliberately and consciously slow and steady your breathing. This sends a message to your body that you are physically feeling calm.
- When you smile, the arrangement of your facial muscles tells your brain you're happy, which can actually make you feel more optimistic: watching a familiar, heart-warming television series or movie can help you relax and switch off for a while.
- Gentle physical exercise (see page 159) stimulates the production of mood-enhancing endorphins, so try 10 minutes of yoga stretches or a gentle walk.
- If you can't get out into nature, even just looking at a picture of a rural landscape, such as trees, hills, a lake or the sky, helps to counteract urban stress.
- Listen to music that resonates with your alpha brain waves This will encourage you to move into a more calm and relaxed state.

24-HOUR CRISIS PLAN: RECAP

- Pay attention to your symptoms. When you spot the signs of burnout, take action fast.
- Look at the list of first steps and commit to following them for at least a day (ideally longer). Clear your diary wherever possible, try to stay off your computer and social media, avoid any potential stressors and try to create a calm environment.
- If burnout is approaching and you can't take these actions, try something from the burnout first aid list to tide you over until you can take a real break.
- Remember, these are just the first steps, and will not be enough to hold burnout at bay in the long term.

06

·

Four Weeks
to Recover
Your Life

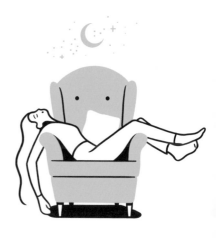

Altering your Baseline

The most important thing to remember is that, once your body has made an adaptation to chronic stress, it has reset its baseline (see page 24) and it will take time to recalibrate. While the 24-hour Crisis Plan (see page 131) can be helpful to alleviate the immediate symptoms of burnout, it is only the beginning of recovery. Remember that it will take time to get the body back into balance: deeply entrenched insomnia won't improve overnight; digestive problems take a while to resolve; knee-jerk reactions that drive heart rate and blood pressure up, and the panicky feelings that result, will take time to settle. That endless underlying anxiety that it's just not possible to get back on top of your life will improve too, but again, it takes *time*. Once your baseline has been altered, there's no point expecting to get back to normal within 24 hours, or a week, or even a month. However, if you are mindful of the changes you need to make in order to avoid or recover from burnout, you will begin to feel different within four weeks.

Keep this in mind and don't panic if you have a good day followed by a less good, or even terrible, one. Allow for a certain amount of fluctuation over this four-week period. Often when we have a good day, we tend to overdo it, and that can create a bit of a lag the following day. If it feels like you're taking two steps forward and one back, remember that this is still progress. Just continue to put one foot in front of the other, taking those positive steps, and it will come together. The secret is not to panic and give up if there's a set-back, but to remind yourself that it just takes time. Remember, too, to ask for help if you need it.

The emphasis here is on taking time to restore and heal, and while this will be individual for everyone stipulating a four-week period reinforces this necessity because when burnout occurs, just taking a break for a short period won't be enough. This four-week programme is only a suggestion and for some it will take much longer to return to their previous baseline.

Week One

Take those emergency steps outlined in the 24-hour crisis plan and review and implement these as necessary every day for the first seven days. Think of this as crisis management and the first stage of a recovery programme.

Week Two

Work towards reinforcing new habits like regular bedtimes (see page 149), gentle exercise, breathing exercises (see page 60) and mindful meditation, which will allow your recovery to take hold and become sustainable over time. Remember to maintain good nutrition and regular mealtimes, gentle exercise, sleep hygiene (see page 146) and time-out from social media, for example.

Week Three

At this point you may feel that your recovery is nearly complete but consider it as a convalescence period and ensure that you're mindful about not over-doing things just because you're beginning to feel better. If you have a bad day, just reinforce some of those steps from week one to get you back on track.

Week Four

This is the point at which newly acquired positive habits should begin to feel well established and you can begin to feel confident about your body's return to a better baseline state. Managing your stress better should become easier for you now you have a set of tools on which you can rely to restore your physical and emotional equanimity.

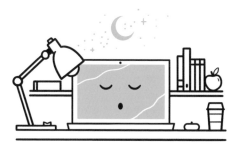

Work Life

It may seem unreasonable to just drop out of work for four weeks, but the truth is you may have to if you have reached peak burnout. If this is the case, the physical impact may force your hand, or your doctor might issue a sick note. If this does happen to you, remember that this time off is for your recuperation and convalescence. This time off is not only in your best interests, but also that of your employer: both productivity and creativity – two key aspects of many working lives – are adversely affected by burnout and this is becoming increasingly recognised and acknowledged. It is also reasonable to use this time to consciously re-evaluate your working life to see how it could be made more manageable in the future and ensure it doesn't threaten your health again.

Even if you don't end up taking a significant amount of time off from work, there are steps you can and should take to improve your work–life balance and keep burnout at bay. UK mental health charity MIND lists various ways to start the process of improving work–life balance.

Are you often the last to leave work?

We know you'll have times when you need to work overtime to meet deadlines, but try to make this the exception, not the norm. The long-hours culture means you may be work harder, but not better and this will quickly take a toll on your concentration, productiveness and health.

Create clear boundaries between work & home

Try not to let work spill over into your personal life. If you need to bring work home, designate a separate area for work and stick to it; you'll find it much easier to then close the door on work.

Start a To-do list

At the end of each day, go over your list and write up one for the next day. When your thoughts are down on paper, you'll find it easier to not think about work.

Use the time on your commute home to wind down from work

Read a book or listen to your music to set aside some time to yourself. Maybe try cycling part of your journey or getting off a stop early to take a shortcut through a park or quiet streets. These little actions can really help you to switch off.

Ask for help

If you feel your workload is spiralling out of control, take the opportunity to discuss it with your manager or supervisor. If you can't resolve the problem of unrealistic goals, organisation problems or deadlines in this way, talk to your personnel department, trade union representative or other relevant members of staff.

'TOP TIPS FOR STAYING WELL AT WORK', MIND

If your workplace has an HR or occupational health department, this may be your first port of call to see what support they may be able to offer you before you take up any concerns with your line manager. Looking after employees' mental health is increasingly being recognised as a priority by many industries and employers.

MANAGING YOUR TIME WHEN YOU'RE NOT AT WORK

It's not only when we're at work that we need to take a step back and decelerate if burnout feels imminent.. Try to manage your time and resources throughout the day. Here are some tips to consider.

◆ Leave gaps in your diary rather than striving to fill every moment with activity. Easing the pressures on your time will help you to slow down.

- Set aside a time of day to turn off all the technology that keeps you buzzing – phones, computers, tablets, television Use the break to sit quietly alone reading a book, listening to music or in mindful meditation.
- Make time for at least one hobby that slows you down, such as reading, painting, gardening or yoga. Use that time to really focus on what you're doing.
- Eat your meals at the table instead of balancing a plate on your lap in front of the television. Take the time to enjoy it, rather than seeing food as mere fuel.
- Try to be aware of and decrease your speed. If you're doing something more quickly than you need to simply out of habit, take a deep breath and slow down.
- Forget FOMO (fear of missing out) and cultivate JOMO (joy of missing out).

SMALL CHANGES

Try to find ways to do things more slowly. Think about tasks that you might usually rush through, like doing the washing up, and try to deliberately perform them more slowly and calmly.

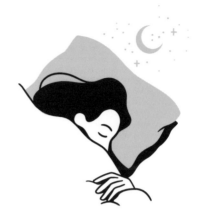

Sleep Well

Sleep is often one of the first casualties of a hyperactive, over-stimulated state of body and mind. A continued lack of sleep will contribute further to the possibility of burnout.

Put simply, our modern lifestyles place great demands on our time, and sleep is often the first thing we sacrifice. We pay a significant price for this.

A tired body demands help to stay awake. A lack of adequate, restorative sleep makes us secrete stress hormones to compensate for chronic fatigue. This in turn makes us feel more stressed and sleep becomes increasingly elusive. Think about how, after a very late night, maybe spent wildly socialising, drinking and dancing, or generally being hyper-stimulated, you might find your heart racing madly the next day. That is the adrenaline effect writ large: a body revved up for action when your mind is saying, *I must rest and recover.*

An occasional lack of sleep can be easily compensated for but, over time, a chronically hyper-stimulated body with an altered baseline (see page 24) finds it increasingly difficult to change modes from switched-on to switched-off. Our capacity to relax, then sleep well or peacefully, is, to put it bluntly, screwed. Chronic fatigue leads to chronic exhaustion.

Before bed

There are steps you can take before you go to bed, some of which also help to provide your body with the 'cues' it needs that it's time to sleep. This is often referred to as 'good sleep hygiene'.

- Avoid *any* caffeine after 3 p.m.
- Avoid any screens, such as laptops, smartphones and tablets, for two hours before bed.
- Eat a light, nutritious supper around four hours before bedtime.
- Avoid over-energetic exercise, but spend 10 minutes doing a gentle stretching and breathing (see page 60) routine.
- Take a warm bath, or ensure your feet are warm before bed, but make sure that the room in which you sleep isn't overheated.

- Have a slow-release carbohydrate-based snack before bed: a milky drink, a banana, or an oat cake with Marmite or avocado (which also contains magnesium, see page 155).
- Avoid over-stimulating news or high-octane entertainment prior to sleep.
- Ensure your bedroom lighting is low key.
- Enjoy an orgasm! The release of anti-stress hormone oxytocin is calming.

To improve your sleep, you also have to review your lifestyle and think about how you spend the 24 hours of each and every day. It's not enough to only focus on the hour or two *before* you go to bed, you also need to consider how you spend the rest of your day, because sleep is part of a 24-hour cycle.

We are diurnal animals. That is, we are designed to be active during the day, when it's light, and to rest and sleep during the night, when it's dark. Depending on where we live in the world, there's a pattern of day and night in each 24 hours. The nearer we are to the equator, the more equal is the length of day and night: 12 hours of light, 12 of dark.

We respond physically to light and darkness. When the eye is exposed to light, the secretion of the sleep hormone melatonin is inhibited. Without its secretion, we tend not to feel sleepy. Dim and darkening light stimulates the secretion of melatonin, and this is a crucial aid to feeling sleepy and falling asleep.

Artificial light allows us to accommodate short daylight hours, but this is often also extended into periods of time that are crucial for sleep. In addition to the artificial lighting we use in our homes, the bright light from our many gadgets – smartphones, laptops, the television – all inhibit the secretion of melatonin. Scrolling through Twitter, checking emails, and sending or reading text messages all contribute to the same effect.

Studies have shown that melatonin can be as effective as benzodiazepine (Valium) in reducing anxiety prior to surgery, so there are no prizes for guessing that its production is calming and therefore an aid to sleep. Melatonin is secreted by the pineal gland in the brain when the level of light entering our eyes diminishes. Our use of bright lights or LED screens is unhelpful prior to sleep because it inhibits the natural melatonin effect. Knowing how to harness your own inbuilt supply of soporific melatonin is important. While we prize good lighting for daytime and work environments, and now opt for many energy saving alternatives, it may be essential to review the lighting levels in your bedroom and make some adjustments if you want to improve your ability to fall asleep.

- Use lights no brighter than a 60-watt bulb or its equivalent in the bedroom.
- Avoid LED and halogen lighting in bedrooms, as these tend to be blue-tinged or white light and too bright.
- Compact fluorescent bulbs also tend to emit blue light so should be avoided in bedrooms.
- Red-tinged light bulbs are most conducive to sleep.

SMALL CHANGES

Try changing the lightbulb in your bedside light to one that's warmly tinted red to help you relax and encourage the secretion of melatonin as you wind down to sleep.

Keep regular hours

This is crucial. Often our sleep patterns become disorganised because we constantly try to sleep and wake at irregular hours: this includes napping and sleeping-in at weekends to try and compensate for our tiredness. Re-setting our internal clock takes time, so make a commitment to go to bed at a regular time every night and set an alarm to wake at the same time every morning. Over the course of a week or two, this will help restore your sleep.

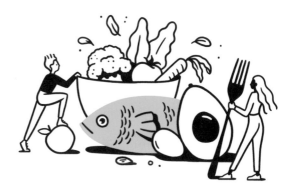

Eat Smart

You may already be aware that your daily diet is poor, or this might be the first time you've ever thought about it. There's no doubt that if you eat a lot of processed foods (including ready-made meals and takeaways), your intake of the nutrients, vitamins and minerals your body needs to stay healthy may be deficient, while your intake of saturated fats, salt and sugar may be too high.

A poor diet cannot give your body what it needs to function well. Poor nutrition can also adversely affect your mood. This doesn't mean that you need to become a food expert or obsessive over what you eat, but it's useful to know the basics of a healthy diet, and aim to stick to this at least 80 per cent of the time if you want to improve your nutritional intake.

Don't underestimate how important diet can be. If you are serious about avoiding or recovering from burnout, improving your daily diet will pay dividends.

Food basics

Our bodies need a balance of protein, carbohydrates and fats from the four main food groups to provide us with what we need. The four main groups are potatoes, rice, cereals and other starchy carbohydrates; meat, fish, eggs, beans and other proteins; dairy products and other fats; and fruit and vegetables.

PROTEIN

Proteins contain the building blocks (amino acids) that help build and repair the body, which we need to keep strong. Protein is also a source of energy. ***Sources:*** *meat, fish, eggs, dairy products, soy products, nuts and pulses.*

Eating protein-rich foods also helps to reduce blood sugar spikes, because protein helps to control the insulin release that is triggered by eating carbohydrates. Eating a bar of chocolate for an energy hit can help, but it will create an insulin surge that your body then has to deal with. It will also leave you feeling hungry again sooner rather than later, so it doesn't provide as sustained an effect as more complex carbohydrates (see page 153).

Protein intake is also important because it provides the amino acids that are crucial building blocks for all body cells, including neurotransmitters – this means it is vital for the biochemical process of thinking. Protein digestion requires adequate micro-nutrients, found in vitamins and minerals, to convert amino acids into neurotransmitters.

CARBOHYDRATES

Carbohydrates can be divided into complex, slow-release, low G.I. (see below) and simple carbohydrates. **Complex sources:** *wholegrains, oats, wholemeal pastas, brown rice.* **Simple sources:** *sugar (sucrose), honey, fruits (fructose) and milk (lactose).*

Our primary source of energy is glucose, derived from carbohydrates digested by the body. What the body likes best is a well-regulated supply, rather than the peaks and troughs that can occur when there are large gaps between eating. This see-sawing effect can also be improved by complex carbohydrates with a low GI (Glycaemic Index – the rate at which carbohydrates are converted into glucose for use by the body). Low G.I. foods have a longer digestive period, and release more consistent levels of glucose more slowly and over a sustained period.

Non-digestible carbohydrates also supply us with dietary fibre, which helps our digestion, and reduces the risk of constipation and other bowel diseases. **Dietary fibre sources:** *fresh fruit and vegetables, wholegrains, beans, pulses, fruit and vegetables.*

FATS

Fats provide energy and essential fatty acids that we can't produce ourselves. They are also a source of fat-soluble vitamins A and D. **Sources:** *animal and vegetable fats, dairy products, oily fish, seeds, avocados.*

Dietary fat comes in a variety of forms: monounsaturated fats, polyunsaturated fats, saturated fats and trans fats (this list ranges from 'good' to 'bad'). Olive oil is an example of a monounsaturated fat, along with avocados. Polyunsaturated fats include omega-3 fatty acids, found in oily fish. Saturated fats come mainly from animal sources such as meat and dairy products. Trans or hydrogenated fats should be completely avoided. They have been officially banned in many countries because they are detrimental to our health and are implicated in obesity, heart disease, cancer and depression.

Vitamins and minerals

A wide variety of foods sourced from the three groups above should provide all the nutrients the body needs. Supplementation (see page 156) is sometimes necessary if our regular diet excludes some components of these food groups or if we have a digestion problem.

A high proportion of fruit and vegetables is recommended because their vitamin and mineral content provides antioxidants that help neutralise the production of free radicals, a by-product of our metabolism that damages body cells, causing illness and ageing. You can see this process of oxidation in action when you slice an apple and the exposure of its damaged surface to oxygen begins to turn it brown. Adding lemon juice, which contains the antioxidant vitamin C, prevents this, which is why it is often added to products as a natural preservative.

Foods to increase your consumption of in an emergency

In addition to eating nutritious meals at regular intervals, there are certain foods that are worth paying special attention to, to help your recovery in the long term.

VITAMIN C

Vitamin C, found in citrus fruits, sweet peppers, kiwi fruit, kale, guava, broccoli, tomatoes and peas, has been shown to be helpful in combatting stress. German researchers tested this by asking 120 people to first give a speech, then work out a hard maths problem.

Those that had been given vitamin C beforehand had lower blood pressure and lower levels of cortisol after the test.

B VITAMINS

There is good evidence that folic acid and vitamins B6 and B12 play a role in the formation of serotonin and other neurotransmitters. Good sources include wholegrain flour, brown rice, oatmeal, eggs, shellfish, poultry, almonds, lentils and leafy green vegetables like spinach and broccoli.

If you have a completely plant-based diet or are vegan, you will need to take a vitamin B12 supplement. Symptoms of deficiency take a while, but these can be serious, starting with fatigue, depression, anxiety, poor memory and numbness or tingling in the hands and feet. Up to a certain stage, symptoms of B12 deficiency are reversible, but some nerve damage can be extreme.

SMALL CHANGES

Oven roast a mix of pumpkin, sunflower, sesame and flax seeds, tossed in a little tamari or soy sauce beforehand, to make a delicious nutritious snack or to add to a salad.

MAGNESIUM

Magnesium is a mineral that is essential for the function of GABA (gamma-aminobutyric acid) in the brain, a neurotransmitter that has a calming effect on the nervous system and muscles. It also supports the body's use of serotonin (see page 43) to create feelings of well-being and relaxation. Good food sources for magnesium include green leafy vegetables, wheat germ, pumpkin seeds and almonds.

OMEGA-3 FATTY ACIDS

They've been dubbed the alternative to Prozac, and with good reason. A double-blind, randomised clinical trial from Tehran University of Medical Sciences found that 1g pharmaceutical grade omega-3 eicosapentaenoic acid (EPA) supplement had an equal therapeutic affect to a 20mg dose of fluoxetine (Prozac) for clinical depression. Studies conducted by the National Institutes of Health in the US found that the omega-3 fatty acids in walnuts keep the stress hormones cortisol and adrenaline in check. Other sources of omega-3s include herring, mackerel and salmon. The anti-inflammatory properties (see page 43) of omega-3s are also helpful in reducing neuroinflammation, which is linked to anxiety and depression.

TRYTOPHAN

Tryptophan works with vitamin B6 to produce serotonin. Foods high in it include poultry, milk, cereal grains, avocados, and pumpkins.

Supplements

The key message about supplements is in their name: they should be used to *supplement* a good diet, not compensate for a poor one. There is a huge market out there for vitamin and mineral supplements, but these should only be considered after first making sure that your diet is as good as you can make it. It is far better to spend your money on the freshest ingredients that you can afford than to spend it on expensive supplements. It is always better to get your nutrients from food, rather than supplements, if you can.

What to avoid

It is worth avoiding alcohol, caffeine and nicotine when you are trying to avoid or recover from burnout. This may not be the best time to go 'cold turkey' on substances on which your body has some reliance, but it is essential that you review your use of them. They may be exacerbating a heightened state of alertness and contributing to insomnia and other symptoms of nervous arousal. It is important that you wean yourself off these substances, even if you have to do so gradually.

ALCOHOL

Alcohol is the most commonly available, socially acceptable intoxicant, but a hangover can make you feel physically jittery and low in mood, while also revving up your stress hormones to compensate. For some, there's a direct correlation between alcohol and depression, too, probably because of its inflammatory effect on the brain.

CAFFEINE

Caffeine is probably the most widely used stimulant in the world. It is present in coffee and some teas, as well as caffeinated soft drinks like cola (which contains 10–50mg) and Red Bull (which contains as much as 80mg). Once in the bloodstream, caffeine makes the nervous system respond as if to a threat, firing things up; the most obvious physical sign of this is a pounding heartbeat. With the body in a state of hyper-arousal, the mind will become more anxious, which exacerbates things further.

NICOTINE

Nicotine makes your body release the stress hormone adrenaline. This activates your SNS (see page 30), making your heart rate increase, your blood pressure rise, and your breathing become rapid and shallow. If you are trying to regulate your body's stress response, nicotine is unhelpful.

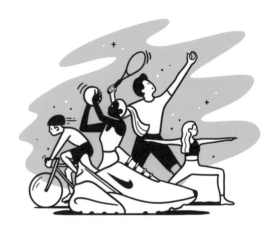

Exercise & Play

When working towards avoiding or recovering from burnout, one way to restore body and mind is through exercise that is fun rather than stress-activating: what can loosely be described as 'play'. You should also consider exercise that includes team-based activities that involve social interaction and positive connection (see page 63) with others.

Exercise

Exercise is the secret weapon of mood enhancement. It works in a number of different ways to increase a feeling of happiness, not just by taking us out of ourselves but also by physically creating mood-enhancing hormones (see page 33) that lift our spirits. Research also suggests that exercise may actually help ward off depression and anxiety by enhancing our natural ability to respond to stress. What's more, it takes relatively little regular exercise to make a big difference to our mood.

Exercise also helps to balance the sympathetic nervous system (SNS) with the parasympathetic nervous system (PNS, see page 30). People who exercise regularly show greater accessibility to their PNS, so it would seem that the more stimulation it receives, the stronger it becomes and the better balanced the two systems are. This helps us manage our stress response.

When we have been through a high-stress period, whether battling through work deadlines or dealing with personal circumstances that are taking their toll, we might bounce back faster if we are more resilient (see page 67). Therefore it really helps to include downtime that switches our focus away from stress-inducing activities, like rumination (see page 57), and towards those that engage us positively in both mind and body, helping to regulate our stress response and restore what baseline (see page 24) is normal for us.

It can be helpful to plan pleasurable activities like exercise ahead of time, so that we can enjoy positively anticipating them before they take place (thinking about future happy events in itself helps soothe brain activity). It's also helpful to use exercise immediately before, or after, a stressful event. For example, if you have to give a presentation at work, taking a brisk walk around the block before or after helps engage a different part of the brain, and the physical process of walking has a positive effect in regulating the stress response.

GET OUTSIDE
Research by Gregory Bratman from Stanford University found that walking through a leafy, quiet, park-like environment had a soothing

effect on the prefrontal cortex of the brain, helpful to reduce the sort of rumination (see page 57) that can lead to anxiety and depression. It also seemed to make those who participated in the study happier and more attentive afterwards, too.

If exercising specifically to help avoid or recover from burnout, it's important that the focus should be on gentle, non-competitive exercise that doesn't induce further stress. For this purpose, avoid high-intensity, stress-inducing activities like running, cardio or weights, and factor in more walking, swimming, dance, yoga or Pilates to restore the body/mind balance.

EXERCISE AND BDNF

Brain-derived neurotrophic factor (BDNF) supports the production of new connections between neurons in the brain and has been dubbed 'Miracle-Gro' because of its effect. During exercise, our muscles produce a protein known as IGF-1 that stimulates the production of BDNF in the brain. Back in 2008, research published in the academic journal *Progress in Neuro-Psychopharmacology and Biological Psychiatry* looked at the connection between BDNF and the HPA axis (see page 25) in the neurobiology of burnout. The researchers concluded that: 'Our results suggest that low BDNF might contribute to the neurobiology of burnout syndrome and it seems to be associated with burnout symptoms including altered mood and cognitive functions.'

Subsequent research in 2019 extensively tested 40 'stress-related exhaustion disorder' patients at the Institute of Stress Medicine in Gothenburg, Sweden, and found that levels of BDNF were significantly lower in this group than in the control group. They also got lower scores for immediate memory, attention and total cognitive function. While other studies have reported that midlife work-related stress and psychological stressors are associated with an increased risk of dementia and Alzheimer's disease, this study also concluded that long-term stress exposure might increase vulnerability to the sort of neurological problems that are being reported today.

For these and other reasons, if you are aiming to restore your life balance and avoid or recover from burnout, daily, moderate exercise must be included in your plan.

Play

Another benefit of play is that it takes our minds off our worries and offers a neurological break from the over-thinking that can contribute to stress. This play can be solitary or with others but should avoid any competitive edge. Focus, instead, on creative activities like drawing or painting, or those that engage our spatial awareness like jigsaw puzzles or are problem solving like crossword puzzles.

Consciously activating the rational brain through play helps with emotional self-regulation which will, in turn, help us when it comes to managing negative emotions and achieving a more balanced response to stressful situations. Emotional self-regulation helps prevent the stress activated freeze/fight/flight response hijacking your body and mind. Anything you do regularly to support the rational brain and improve self-regulation will support you in avoiding or recovering from burnout.

SMALL CHANGES

Put a calming, logic-based game app on your smartphone and try to play that rather than scrolling through social media.

SHARED ACTIVITIES

Because connectedness, in real life, does so much to enhance our well-being, it can be good to share other activities as well as exercise. Socialising and having fun with those we care about is an essential part of restoring balance. Whether this is a sharing a meal, playing a board game, watching a movie or television show together or taking a walk, it all helps to maintain those connections that are so important to our well-being.

FOUR WEEKS TO RECOVER YOUR LIFE: RECAP

- Take some time off work if you can and set clear boundaries to improve your work–life balance.
- Make an effort to slow down outside work, too.
- Sleep is a key factor. Learn to manage your environment, devices and routine to aid better sleep.
- Eat well. Make sure you are getting the vitamins and minerals your body needs to function, and learn which foods and substances to avoid.
- Daily, moderate exercise creates mood-enhancing hormones and relieves stress. Team sports offer you a chance to connect with others.
- Make time to play, whether alone or with friends.
- Remember that this is going to take time. Keep going, and you will begin to see progress.

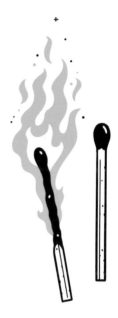

Conclusion: From Burnout to Balance

Burnout is better avoided than experienced. Keep it at bay by:

◆ being smart to your own indicators of stress, managing them and avoiding their escalation by making lifestyle changes;

◆ ensuring you take basic self-care measures every day – adequate sleep, regular nutritious meals, exercise and relaxation – to keep your body and mind resilient;

* saying no to excessive demands on your time;
* asking for help when it's needed;
* creating a support system;
* relinquishing perfection.

These are the behaviours of confident people who know that before you help anyone else with their oxygen mask, you must first fit your own.

Remember: if a high-performance car is driven relentlessly at full throttle and burnout occurs, it doesn't just falter to a gradual stop; all systems fail.

BURNOUT TO BALANCE: FULL RECAP
Understanding the signs
* Learn to recognise the warning signs of burnout, including emotional, physical and mental exhaustion, a sense of being cut off from friends, colleagues and the world around you, and a feeling of being ineffective at whatever you're doing.

Understanding stress
* Our bodies don't differentiate between emotional and physical trauma, so emotional stress can have a physical impact
* Subjecting ourselves to relentless stress means our bodies are unable to return to a healthy 'baseline' state.
* Functioning at a perpetual level of red alert is damaging to both our psychological and physical health.
* Many of us breathe shallowly without realising, which creates

a stress reaction in the body. Learning to breathe deeply enables us to calm and control this reaction. You can also practice mindfulness meditation, which focuses on the breath.

* Working to increase our resilience and understand what we can and can't control can help us to become better at dealing with stress.
* If you're struggling with feeling overwhelmed or overworked, ask for help.

The effects of work and social media

* Workplace stressors, like long hours, high pressure and a poor physical and emotional environment can all contribute to burnout.
* Pay attention to the things (and possibly people) at work that make you feel stressed, and consider what options are available to you in terms of addressing these issues.
* Even though social media is supposed to be (and can be) fun, we need to pay close attention to how we use it and how it makes us feel. Sometimes spending time on social media can actually make us feel more isolated.
* Switching between lots of different platforms and apps can make us feel overwhelmed and lead to Continuous Partial Attention (CPA).
* Recognise when it's time to take a break from scrolling.

When burnout hits: 24-hour crisis plan

* Take action fast. Clear your diary, turn off your social media accounts and try to avoid any potential stressors.
* Rest as much as possible.

- Eat small amounts of nutritious, easy-to-prepare foods at regular intervals.
- Try some very gentle exercise, like a slow walk or some yoga stretches.

When burnout hits: 4-week recovery plan

- If you can, take some time off work and use this opportunity to consider the sort of boundaries you might need to implement to improve your work–life balance.
- Make an effort to slow down outside work, too.
- Learn how to create the right environment for restful sleep, which is vital for recovery.
- Exercise releases feel-good hormones like endorphins and serotonin, which will help to balance out stress. Exercise regularly, but moderately – avoid high-stress exercise like running or very competitive sports. Opt for swimming, yoga and low-pressure team sports.
- Make sure you're eating well. Try to incorporate anti inflammatory foods as well as all the vitamins and minerals you need to nourish your body.
- Be kind to yourself. Take your time. Keep breathing.
- Spend more time in natural surroundings, walking, gardening or just enjoying a changing or peaceful view.

Acknowledging that you are in the throes of burnout can be scary and overwhelming, but taking the steps outlined in this book will support your recovery. Remember that this takes time, however, so be patient with yourself as you return to a place of balance.

Appendix

Further reading

- *Healing Without Freud or Prozac*, Dr David Servan-Schreiber (Rodale, 2004)
- *Stress Proof: The Ultimate Guide to Living a Stress-Free Life*, Dr Mithu Storoni (Yellow Kite, 2019
- *The Body Keeps the Score: Mind, Brain and Body in the Transformation of Trauma*, Bessel van der Kolk (Penguin Books, 2014)
- *The Energy Book*, Richard Maddocks (LID Publishing Ltd, 2019)
- *The Inflamed Mind*, Edward Bullmore (Short Books, 2018)
- *The Joy of Burnout*, Dina Glouberman (Skyros Books, 2002)
- *The Well-Gardened Mind: Rediscovering Nature in the Modern World*, Sue Stuart-Smith (Harper Collins, 2020)
- *Thrive*, Arianna Huffington (WH Allen, 2014)

Useful Websites

- Calm.com
- Headspace.com
- Mind.org.uk
- Mindandlife.org
- Mindtools.com
- Plumvillage.org
- Welldoing.org

About the Author

Harriet Griffey is an internationally-respected writer and journalist, focusing much of her work on health. She originally trained and worked as a state registered nurse in the UK, is an accredited coach and stress counsellor, and has published over thirty health-related titles including the bestselling *I Want to...* series for Hardie Grant.

Acknowledgements

Any book on a subject like this relies on the work of many, so I'd like to acknowledge all the psychologists, physiologists and other scientists who have researched burnout over the years and contributed so much to our understanding of this peculiarly contemporary phenomenon and what we can do about it.

In addition, I'd also like to thank my editor Eve Marleau and the team at Hardie Grant publishers, particularly Kate Pollard, Kajal Mistry and Eila Purvis. It's a real pleasure to work alongside their talent, industry and good humour. My thanks are also due to designer Julia Murray, who always brings the benefit of her creative talents to my books with such flair.

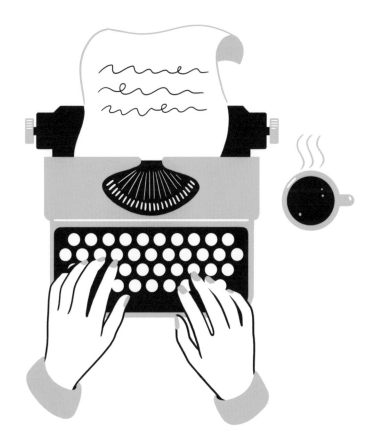

Index

activities, shared 163
adrenal glands 12, 20, 25
adrenaline 12, 25, 33, 40, 55, 60, 63, 109, 146, 156, 157
alcohol 156–7
alpha brain waves 130, 131
amygdala 30
antioxidants 42–3, 154
anxiety 39, 127, 136
  and emotional self-regulation 110
  exercise and 159
  medication 84
  melatonin and 148
  omega-3 fatty acids and 156
  rumination and 161
  social isolation and 64
  uncertainty and 71
apps 115, 116, 163, 167
atrial fibrillation (AF) 14
autonomic nervous system (ANS) 30, 55

balance: first steps to 129–31
  recovery plan 132–63
  work-life balance 140
baseline: altered 24, 146
  normal 11, 24, 160, 166
  resetting your 135–7
baths 130, 146
biophilia 78–9
blood pressure 56, 63, 135, 155, 157
the brain: brain fog 25
  rewiring 77–8
brain-derived neurotrophic factor (BDNF) 78, 161–2
Bramson, Dr Robert 98
Bratman, Gregory 160–1

breaks, taking 94, 95
breathing: breathing exercises 57, 59–61, 130, 131, 137
  shallow breathing 59–60, 166–7
bullies 99, 113
Bullmore, Edward 110
burnout: 24-hour crisis plan 122–31, 135, 167
  avoiding 165–8
  burnout quiz 47–51
  identifying the problem 23–6
  long-term impact of 15
  Maslach Burnout Inventory (MBI) 11
  pandemic-induced 7–8
  signs & symptoms of 10, 11–12, 13, 16–51, 125, 127, 166
  when to ask for help 81–5
  WHO definition 9–10, 13, 15

caffeine 127, 130, 146, 156–7
carbohydrates 41, 152, 153
catastrophising 69
central nervous system 34
chronic fatigue 15, 146
cognitive behavioural therapy (CBT) 78, 83
colleagues 97–9
commutes 141
continuous partial attention (CPA) 109–10, 167
coronavirus 7–8
cortisol 12, 25, 33, 40, 55, 60, 63, 109, 156

counselling 83
creativity 9, 140, 162
crisis plan, 24-hour 122–31, 135, 167

depression 11, 39
  alcohol and 157
  CBT and 83
  and emotional self-regulation 110
  exercise and 159
  medication 34, 84
  omega-3 fatty acids 156
  rumination and 161
  serotonin and 34
  social isolation and 64
diet 129, 137, 151–7, 165, 168
Dines, Christopher 72, 76
discontent, social media and 113
dopamine 35
downtime 84, 141, 160

EMDR (eye movement desensitisation reprogramming) 84
emotions 127, 162
endorphins 34, 40, 131, 168
environment, workplace 93–5
exercise 84, 137, 159–62
  and BDNF 78, 161–2
  calming 129, 161
  and endorphins 34, 40, 131, 168
  mindful 78
  pre-bed 146
  and stress hormones 40
exhaustion 20, 25, 127
expectations, workplace 101–3

fatigue 15, 25, 146
fats 152, 153–4
fertility problems 15
fibre 153
fight/flight/freeze response 25, 30, 55, 60, 162
Firestone, Lisa 77
FOMO (fear of missing out) 142
food 151–7, 165, 168
  foods to avoid 156–7
  foods to increase 41–3, 152–6
free radicals 42, 154

GABA 155
gardening 79
Garg, Dr Parveen 14, 25
genes, our well-being and 34–5
gig economy 14, 90
glucose 153
Glycaemic Index (GI) 153
group therapy 83–4

habits, reinforcing new 137
happiness, baseline level of 35
heart problems 14, 127, 135
help, asking for 81–5, 136, 141, 166, 167
hippocampus 30
hobbies 142
hormones, feel-good 33–6
Horta-Osorio, António 8–9
HPA axis 25, 161
hugs 36, 63
hurtful words 31

hydration 130
hyperventilation 59–60
hypothalamus 25, 30

immune system 15
inflammation 39–44, 110, 157
insomnia 25, 135, 157
Institute of Stress Medicine 161–2
isolation 12, 107, 167

JOMO (joy of missing out) 142
judging yourself or others 77

Leiter, Professor Michael 68
life-work balance 140
limbic system 29–31, 120
loneliness 64
lunch breaks 94, 95

maladaptation 24
Maslach Burnout Inventory (MBI) 11
medication 34, 84
meditation 61, 76, 137, 167
melatonin 147, 148
micro-interruptions 109
millennials 12
MIND 140, 141
mindfulness: meditations 76, 137, 167
  mindful living 75–9
  mindfulness-based cognitive therapy 83
minerals 154, 155, 156, 168
multitasking 13–14, 77
music 130, 131, 141
Myers, Benjamin 24

nature 78–9, 131, 160–1, 168
negativity 113, 119, 120
Neve, Jan-Emmanuel de 35
news 119, 120, 130, 147
nicotine 156–7
omega-3 fatty acids 42, 153, 156
optimism 131
outdoor environments 78–9, 131, 160–1, 168
overtime 140
oxidation 42, 154
oxytocin 36, 63, 147

pandemic-induced burnout 7–8
parasympathetic nervous system (PNS) 30, 55, 56, 57, 130, 160
personality types 98
perspective, sense of 69
Pichai, Sundar 7
pituitary gland 25, 34
play 159, 162–3
post-traumatic stress disorder (PTSD) 84
processed foods 151
productivity 9, 55, 90, 140
protein 41, 152
psychotherapy 83
recovery plan 132–63, 168
relationships 63–4, 91, 159
repetitive strain injury 94
resilience 47, 67–9, 160, 167
rumination 57, 72, 75, 78, 83, 161
Sandburg, Sheryl 8
screen time 115–16, 146

sedentary lifestyles 40–1, 94
self-acceptance 77
self-care 125, 165
self-esteem 107
self-help 84
serotonin 34, 155, 156, 168
sex 147
sick days 55, 91
sleep 84, 127, 165
  bedtimes 137
  insomnia 11, 25, 135, 157
'snowflake' generation 11, 12, 67
social media 64, 104–21, 129, 137, 163, 167
Stone, Linda 109
stress: being stress smart 52–85
  chronic 15, 120, 135
  continuous low-level 20, 23–4, 71
  definition of 54–7
  exercise and 160
  expectations and 102–3
  and fertility 15
  how to manage 39, 56
  inflammation and 39–40
  personal stress responses 56
  sleep and 146
  social media 104–21
  understanding 166–7
  workplace 86–103
stress hormones 11, 12, 20, 40
  alcohol and 157
  effect of the news on 120
  exercise and 40
  and fertility 15

the heart and 127
  hyper-alert state 109–10
  sleep and 146
stretches 94, 146
supplements 43–4, 154, 156
sympathetic nervous system (SNS) 30, 55, 56, 57, 157, 160

Takotsubo cardiomyopathy 31
talking treatments 82–4
therapy 78, 83–4
time management 115, 116, 141–2
time out, taking 9
to-do lists 140
tryptophan 156

uncertainty 71–3, 91

vagus nerve 56, 57, 130
vitamins 154–5, 156, 168

work and workplaces 89–91
  colleagues 97–9
  environment 93–5
  expectations 101–3
  home working 7–8
  mental health provisions 82, 90
  work life 139–42
  workplace stress 86–103, 167
World Health Organisation 9–10, 13, 15
worry 69, 72, 78
young people, social media and 113

Published in 2020 by Hardie Grant Books,
an imprint of Hardie Grant Publishing

Hardie Grant Books (London)
5th & 6th Floors
52–54 Southwark Street
London SE1 1UN

Hardie Grant Books (Melbourne)
Building 1, 658 Church Street
Richmond, Victoria 3121

hardiegrantbooks.com

British Library Cataloguing-in-Publication Data. A catalogue record
for this book is available from the British Library.

From Burnout to Balance by Harriet Griffey

ISBN: 978-1-78488-362-1

10 9 8 7 6 5 4 3 2 1

Publishing Director: Kate Pollard
Senior Editor: Eve Marleau
Design and Illustrations: Julia Murray
Editor: Tara O'Sullivan
Proofreader: Sarah Herman
Indexer: Vanessa Bird

Colour reproduction by p2d
Printed and bound in China by Leo Paper Products Ltd.

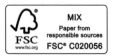